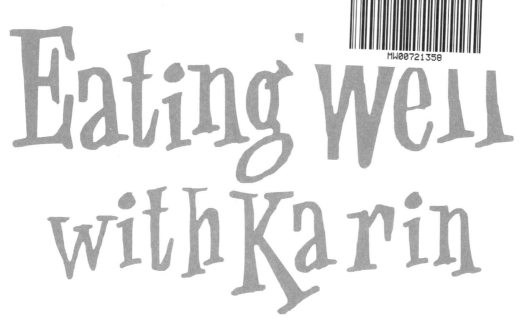

Eating Well with Karin

Recipes for Every Body

Karin Laronde Antolick

The Acorn Press
Charlottetown
2012

To Marion & Ernest: Eat Well! Love from Karin

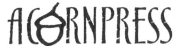

P.O. Box 22024
Charlottetown, Prince Edward Island
C1A 9J2
acornpresscanada.com

Printed and Bound in Canada
Design by Matt Reid
Cover photography by John Sylvester Photography
Editing by Caitlin Drake

Library and Archives Canada Cataloguing in Publication

Antolick, Karin Laronde
      Eating well with Karin : recipes for every
body / Karin Laronde Antolick.

Includes index.
ISBN 978-1-894838-90-0

      1. Cooking. 2. Health--Nutritional aspects. 3. Nutrition.
4. Cookbooks. I. Title.

RA784.A59 2012   641.5'63   C2012-905667-7

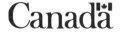 Canada Council for the Arts Conseil des Arts du Canada

The publisher acknowledges the support of the Government of Canada through the Canada Book Fund of the Department of Canadian Heritage and the Canada Council for the Arts Block Grant Program.

MARION

Dedicated to Mom and Dad

Table of Contents

Foreword

I first met Karin at the Bonnie Brae Restaurant, which I co-owned, where she worked for many years. What I most remember about her during those times was her great attitude towards food, and the smiles she had to share with our customers. She was always happy to help in any way.

Years later, her passion took her to a new adventure when she enrolled at the Culinary Institute in the Hospitality Program. I was then an instructor there when our paths crossed again. After graduating she started a business at home and also was selling at the Farmers Market in Charlottetown where I was a regular customer. Whenever we met, it always a pleasure chatting with her. She always used fresh local products as much as possible, even buying some of my chanterelle mushrooms.

It's a joy to see that she's decided to put all her energy and knowledge into this wonderful cook book. Inside you'll find really useful information on ingredients and equipment she used. There are also many healthy and delicious gluten free and vegan recipes, as well as a number of helpful tips.

I hope this book inspires you to appreciate food the way Karin does.

- Hans Anderegg

Hans Anderegg is a Chef Instructor at the Culinary Institute of Canada.

Getting to Know Me

Greetings!

Thank you for taking an interest in this cookbook. This book has been a project of love for me, and I believe you will find numerous recipes that you will enjoy within its pages. Many of the recipes are perfect to serve to your family, but there are quite a few that are company or potluck worthy, as well. (Those are the ones that get you invited to more potlucks!)

I have always taken an interest in cooking and started in the food industry while I was a teenager. I worked in restaurants as a waitress, then as a maître d'hotel, all the while observing the talented chefs I worked alongside and their culinary practices. I later received some formal chef training of my own at the Culinary Institute of Canada while I was taking the Hospitality Management Program at Holland College in Charlottetown.

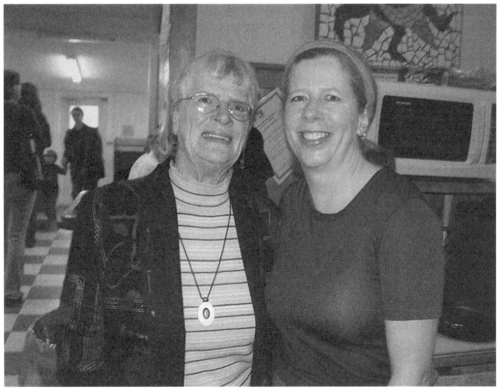

My mother was an excellent cook, so I'm grateful to have received some of her genes.

In 1999, I was stuck for a job, so my friend Sue suggested that I start a catering service. We were finding that there was a need for healthy and nutritious prepared meals for busy people, especially those with dietary requirements such as gluten-free, vegan, vegetarian, low fat, etc.

So, with that vision, I set out small. I'd cook a variety of meals, package and label them, put them in coolers, go to businesses, and attempt to "sell my wares." I was also lucky enough to secure a booth at the Charlottetown Farmers' Market at the same time. I called my business "Eat Well: Food with Thought."

Well, the timing was right, because the business took off. People were becoming more aware of what they were eating and were looking for healthier choices, and there I was with those healthy (and tasty) choices.

The business expanded to catering functions. We catered to workshops, dinner meetings, dinner parties, weddings, and movie and TV sets, all the time still offering the home and business catering delivery twice a week and running our booth at the farmers' market.

During my time in the Eat Well kitchen, I met some of the greatest people I've ever known, many of whom are still a big part of my life today. But the best person I met was my husband, Mike. He was the valiant knight who came on his white horse (i.e. van) and saved the beautiful princess (i.e. stressed-out cook with a broken stove trying to pull off a catering function). He fixed the stove and saved the day, and we lived happily ever after.

In the spring of 2008, I was diagnosed with a rare type of cancer, adenoid cystic carcinoma. I had extensive surgery and received numerous radiation treatments, but in the winter of 2009 my doctors discovered that the cancer had metastasized to both of my lungs, leaving me without treatment options.

I thought it would be best to sell my business and attend to my life. This is not a sad story, though. Surprisingly, at the time I'm writing this it has been more than three years since that diagnosis. And since that diagnosis, I have had a blast! I have been travelling, spending lots of time with my people, totally enjoying my life, realizing the importance of this life, and appreciating every day. I'm still living happily ever after!

Around Christmas of 2011, at a gathering where I brought my famous "How to Get Invited to a Christmas Party" Squares, my friends Janice and Sue (the same Sue who got me started with the business) suggested that I write this cookbook and offer you some of the best recipes we worked with in the Eat Well kitchen. The recipes aren't all mine. Many are, but I've had a lot of great hands in the kitchen who have also contributed, and some of the recipes were found in magazines or online and were changed to my liking.

Mike is getting a kick out of me writing a cookbook, since I'm not one to follow recipes—I like to play around with recipes and change them to suit my tastes. I encourage you to do the same. These recipes are good (great, in fact), but feel free to make them your own. Have fun with them, and enjoy!

Blessings,
Karin

Getting Started

In this chapter we have included some tips and ideas for you, whether you are a kitchen rookie or have plenty of cooking hours under your belt. Perhaps the answer to one of those queries that you have always wondered about is in this chapter, such as what to do with the package of tofu that has been in your fridge for a week, which oils work best for certain cooking methods, or what is the best way to roast vegetables.

in My Pantry

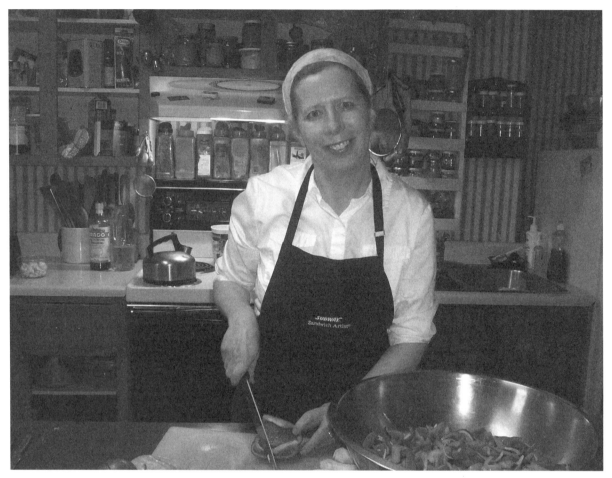

Having a pantry well stocked with non-perishable items and time-saving equipment is the key to quick and easy healthy meals, cooking on the fly, and improvising. Here are my top twenty-one favourite pantry items. What's in your pantry?

FOOD ITEMS

Balsamic Vinegar

Balsamic vinegar is a reduction made from the unfermented must of Trebbiano grapes. You will find a variety of balsamic vinegars in your local stores. Some are worth their high price and others are not. Often, the less expensive ones may suit your needs just fine. Balsamic vinegar is great for salad dressings, dips for vegetables and bread, sauces, and marinades.

Bragg Liquid Aminos

If I were stranded on a desert island and were permitted to have just ten items, one of those items would be Bragg Liquid Aminos. Bragg's robust flavour adds richness to most savoury dishes. It contains natural salt, so be careful to reduce the amount of sea salt if you're going to incorporate it into your dishes. Bragg's is made of non-genetically modified soybeans and water, and it is not fermented. It contains sixteen essential and non-essential amino acids in naturally occurring amounts. Best of all, it is gluten-free. You will see it often in my recipes. You should be able to find Bragg's in health food stores or in the health food section of most large supermarkets with the other condiments.

Brown Lentils

The brown lentil is by far the most common variety of lentil. It is stocked in most local grocery stores. Brown lentils generally have a mild earthy flavour. They cook in 20 to 30 minutes and hold their shape very well. You can use brown lentils in many dishes, including Mjadra (page 116), West Indian Lentil and Cheddar Rotis (page 123), or our very popular Lentil Tourtière (page 124).

Chickpeas (also known as garbanzo beans)

Chickpeas are versatile, full of nutrients, and low in fat. They can be eaten cold in salads, cooked in soups and stews, added to grain or pasta dishes, or ground into flour. Chickpea hummus is great as a dip or as a spread for sandwiches or wraps. It can also be roasted, spiced, and eaten as a snack.

Extra Virgin Olive Oil

This is the highest-quality type of olive oil, characterized by fine flavour and aroma. It contains no more than 0.8% acidity. Extra virgin olive oil is used in salad dressings, served at the table with bread for dipping, or added to soups and stews.

Fresh Garlic

It wasn't until I left home that I first sampled fresh garlic. Prior to that, I thought that all garlic was powdered and came in bottles. There is no doubting that fresh garlic is vastly superior to the bottled variety in both taste and health benefits. Researchers believe that fresh garlic can bolster the immune system, lower blood pressure, and prevent heart disease. Some people even believe that it can ward off insects and vampires! It's perfect in stir-fries and curries, but one of my favourite ways to use it is to roast it. Keep some roasted garlic in your fridge and use it for salad dressings, pastas, or spreading on yummy crusty bread.

Fresh Ginger

Ginger is a powerful spice used in many dishes. You can find this tan, knobby root in the fresh produce aisle. Look for pieces with smooth, thin peels. Due to its powerful taste, most recipes will require you to grate fresh ginger before adding it to a dish or marinade. You can use a microplane or rasp to do this, but I sometimes just chop it finely or pop it into my running food processor. A Chinese friend of mine recommends leaving the peel on for cooking, as long as it is thin and tender. She also suggests storing fresh ginger in a basket at room temperature rather than in the fridge. I've done that for the last three years with great results. If you wish to peel your ginger, try peeling it with a spoon—it's surprisingly efficient.

Green Lentils

The green lentil is a delicate, peppery-flavoured variety originating from Puy, France, but now grown in North America and Italy. Green lentils are approximately 3/16-inch in size and have outer skins that are deep green with dark speckles and interiors that are yellow. Green lentils generally take the longest to cook, upwards of 45 minutes, but they keep a firm texture even after cooking. This makes them ideal for salads and other side dishes.

Quinoa (pronounced KEEN-wa)

Quinoa is one of my favourite grains. It contains essential amino acids like lysine and good quantities of calcium, phosphorus, and iron. The Incas, who held the crop to be sacred, referred to quinoa as "the mother of all grains." Quinoa is generally cooked the same way as rice and can be used in a wide range of dishes. Try using quinoa in our Quinoa and Sweet Potato Maple Salad (page 52) or Toasted Tofu and Quinoa Casserole (page 82).

Red Lentils

The red lentil is the sweetest and nuttiest of the lentils. Red lentils usually take about 30 minutes to cook. They tend to get mushy when cooked through, so they're perfect for Indian dahls and curries or for thickening soups and stews.

Saffron

This rather expensive Spanish spice turns a tasty dish into a fabulous dish. I highly recommend that you keep some in your pantry. Perhaps you could put it on your birthday or Christmas wish list and then invite the gifter over for dinner. Saffron is delicious in paella or aioli

Toasted Sesame Oil

Just a few drops of toasted sesame oil can add an outrageously delicious flavour that enhances many foods. The toasted sesame seeds it's made from give this oil its intense aromatic quality and wonderful robust flavour. Use it when you want an Asian flair. Because it has a low smoke point, it's best to add this oil towards the end of the cooking preparation or to use it in salad dressings.

Tofu

The two types of tofu are regular tofu, which comes in plastic packages, and silken tofu, which comes in aseptic boxes. We always keep two packages of regular tofu in our fridge because most regular tofu has an expiry date of a couple of weeks. When I'm wondering what to cook for supper, the tofu is always in the fridge and ready to go.

There are many ways to serve regular tofu (you will find even more after reading this book) and most of them don't require a lot of preparation. Silken tofu is also great to have on hand. It lasts a long time and you can use it for everything from salad dressings to sauces to desserts.

EQUIPMENT

Food Processor

I honestly don't know how the pioneers prepared meals without a food processor. As you will see in my recipes, I'm quite dependent on this machine. The food processor is excellent for making dips like hummus and tapenade and also for mincing garlic and/or ginger. You can slice the potatoes for Potatoes Anna Karinina (page 58) in seconds or grate the zucchini for Herb and Cheese Zucchini Bread (page 185) in no time. Put it on your wish list if you don't have one.

Hand Blender

This is a very handy tool. I love that I can use it to blend hot items right in the pot, like when I'm puréeing soups. It can also be used for mixing smoothies, batters, and eggs.

Microplane

This is a wonderful tool for a variety of grated items, including hard cheeses, chocolate, nutmeg, cinnamon, and citrus zests. The microplane is extremely easy to use because you can grate right into the pot or onto a plate.

Pepper Mill with Whole Peppercorns

Whole peppercorns that have been freshly ground with a pepper mill deliver more flavour than pre-ground pepper. This is because grinding pepper releases the flavourful volatile oils within, but these oils evaporate after time. The best way to get the full flavour out of your peppercorns is by grinding it directly onto your food at the end of cooking or when serving.

Rice Cooker

I love my rice cooker! It frees up a burner on my stove and it knows how to cook any kind of rice better than I do. It seems to know the difference between brown and white rice and even quinoa. Highly recommended and not too expensive.

Sea Salt Grinder

This tool allows you to freshly grind your own sea salt, which is often too coarse to use directly in dishes. Sea salt is preferable to table salt because it is produced through evaporation of seawater, usually with little processing. This leaves behind certain trace minerals and elements, depending on its water source. Table salt is mined from underground salt deposits. It is more heavily processed, which eliminates minerals, and usually contains an additive to prevent clumping.

Timer

If I didn't have my three cooking timers, everything I make would burn. No matter how conscious I try to be of timing—whether it is 1 minute or 60 minutes—I still need a timer as a reminder.

Yogurt Maker

One of my best flea market finds is my 2-litre yogurt incubator. Every week, I make soy milk yogurt for my husband and regular milk yogurt for me. It is invaluable to me.

Oil Speak

Canada's Food Guide says that we should include a small amount—30 to 45 ml (2 to 3 tbsp.)— of unsaturated fat in our diets each day to get the fat we need. This amount includes oil used for cooking, salad dressings, margarine, and mayonnaise.

TIPS FOR COOKING WITH OIL

- Cooking at high temperatures can damage some oils. The more omega-3 fatty acids in the oil, the less suitable it is for cooking. The heat not only damages the fatty acids, it can also change them into harmful substances. The best oils for cooking at high temperatures are refined peanut, safflower, and sunflower oils.

- The oil or fat you use for frying should have a high smoke point—the temperature to which it can be heated without smoking. Butter has a low smoke point, so it's not good for high-temperature frying, but it will work for light sautéing.

- Unrefined cooking oils are best used for salad dressings, marinades, sauces, light sautés, and low-heat baking. As a general rule, they should not be cooked at high temperatures.

Below are some types of oil and their best uses.

Type	Dressings	Baking	High Smoke Point
Almond	yes	yes	yes
Avocado	yes	yes	yes
Butter	no	yes	no
Coconut	no	yes	no
Extra Virgin Olive*	yes	no	no
Flaxseed	yes	no	no
Grapeseed (refined)	yes	yes	yes
Hazelnut	yes	no	no
Light or Pure Olive **	yes	yes	yes
Peanut (refined)	yes	yes	yes
Safflower (refined)	yes	yes	yes
Sesame (refined)	yes	yes	yes
Sesame (toasted)	yes	no	no
Sunflower (refined)	yes	yes	yes
Walnut	yes	no	no

*Extra virgin olive oil has a strong flavour and may not be good in baking.

**Light or pure olive oil has a higher smoke point than extra virgin olive oil.

TIPS FOR BUYING AND STORING OIL

- If you are buying oil in large quantities, it should be stored in dark bottles. Clear glass or plastic bottles allow light to penetrate the oil and oxidize the fatty acids. If the oil comes in a clear bottle, wrap it with a dark covering.

- Screw the lid of your oil bottle on tightly between uses, because contact with air will affect the quality of the oil.

- Purchase oil in small quantities, and use it within a month or two. The higher-quality oils tend to spoil quicker.

- Store oils in a cool, dark place. Unrefined oils spoil more easily when exposed to warm temperatures, so they need to be refrigerated if you are not going to use them right away. An exception to this is olive oil, which doesn't need refrigeration. It is high in oleic acid and contains antioxidants that slow spoiling. Other cooking oils, such as safflower, sunflower, and corn oil, are high in linolenic acid and are quick to spoil.

How to Make Stock

Stock is the foundation of cooking. It is the base for soups and sauces. It is what we use to stew, braise, and thin liquids and purées. It also adds great flavour and nutrients to your dishes.

In the Eat Well kitchen, we find a use for everything. When peeling and chopping vegetables or herbs, we save the peels and ends and keep them in a bag in the freezer. When we have 4 to 5 cups of peelings, we are ready to make stock.

Here is the recipe we use to make stock using scraps from vegetables.

- **4 to 5 cups vegetable peels and ends***
- **leftover chicken or beef bones****
- **12 cups fresh cold water**
- **3 to 4 bay leaves**
- **10 to 12 black peppercorns**

1. Place all the ingredients in a large pot. Bring the mixture to a boil and then let simmer for 20 to 25 minutes. Don't leave it longer because stock may turn bitter.

2. Strain the vegetables, reserving the liquid. If the liquid looks and tastes flavourful, it is ready to use. If not, you can boil the strained stock until it is reduced to the flavour you want.

*We use scraps from carrots, celery, fresh parsley, fresh thyme, leeks, and onions (which darken the stock). We don't use potato, sweet potato, or broccoli scraps because we find that their flavours are too strong.

**If we want to make beef or chicken stock, we add leftover bones to the recipe. For vegetable stock, we leave the bones out.

The Tricks of Tofu

Tofu has been a large part of Asian cuisine for hundreds of years. Recently it has become popular in Western vegetarian cooking as a replacement for meat. It is a staple in our house.

Tofu is made from soybeans, water, and a coagulant or curdling agent. It is high in protein and calcium and well known for its ability to absorb the flavours from spices and marinades. We buy firm tofu for stir-fries and silken tofu for desserts, smoothies, and sauces. Silken tofu usually comes in aseptic boxes, which give it a long shelf life.

When cooking with firm tofu, drain and press the tofu before using it. To do this, rinse it under cold water and then press it between two small cutting boards in the sink, elevated on a slant so the liquid drains downwards. Place a cloth on the top cutting board and set a cast iron frying pan on top of it to help press the tofu. Leave this for an hour or so. Once the tofu has finished draining, you are ready to cut it up for the recipe.

Tofu has a lot of water in it and acts like a sponge even after you press it. If you're planning on marinating your tofu, it is best not to put oil in your marinade to prevent the tofu from getting too greasy. Vinegars, Bragg's sauce, soy sauce, citrus juice, and seasonings are all terrific tofu marinade ingredients.

If you're planning to use your tofu in a soup or stew, you can preserve the taste of your marinated tofu by frying it in a little oil before adding it to the liquid. This prevents the flavours from tofu from mixing into the soup or stew broth.

SOME IDEAS FOR USING TOFU:

- **Barbecue it. Marinate it for a few hours or overnight and then barbecue it for 4 to 5 minutes on each side.**

- **Bake it. Slice pressed and drained firm tofu blocks into thin strips, marinate it, and then bake it on a cookie sheet (sprayed with nonstick spray) at 350°F for 15 minutes, or until golden brown.**

- **Sauté it. Fry cubes or thin triangles of pressed, drained, and marinated firm tofu in oil until golden brown.**

- **Deep-fry it. Drop thin slices of pressed and drained firm tofu in your deep fryer and cook until light brown and crispy.**

- **Stir-fry it. Sauté chunks of pressed and drained firm tofu much as you would any other meat, then add your favourite stir-fry sauce. The tofu will absorb the flavours of the stir-fry oils and sauce nicely.**

- **Put it in a chili or stew. Add pressed and crumbled firm tofu to chili or stew and cook through for at least 15 minutes at medium heat.**

- **Make it into cheesecake or custard. Replace cream cheese with tofu in cheesecake and custard recipes to create delicious, high-protein desserts.**

- **Make it into a smoothie. Place silken tofu, fresh fruit and/or berries, soy milk, and ice into a blender and blend until smooth for a healthy, protein-laden smoothie.**

Did you know that tofu is an ancient food that was discovered around 164 BC? And also that it is used at Buddhist banquets to imitate meat?

How to Roast or Grill Vegetables and Fruit

The process of roasting or grilling brings out the natural sweetness in vegetables and intensifies their natural flavours. Try roasting a vegetable you thought you weren't fond of—you might get a nice surprise!

Grilled or roasted vegetables can be used in many ways: to accompany fish, beef, or chicken; added to marinated tofu for a complete meal; in a pita or wrap; on pizza; in a salad; in an antipasto platter; or in a vegetarian lasagna. The possibilities are endless!

Winter vegetables such as beets, carrots, potatoes, parsnips, onions, Brussels sprouts, winter squash, and sweet potatoes are perfect for roasting, while spring and summer vegetables such as asparagus, peppers, eggplant, zucchini, fennel, and corn are splendid for grilling.

Most vegetables cook better and are less likely to stick to the pan if tossed with marinade or brushed lightly with cooking oil before grilling or roasting. Marinades are easy to make. Just combine one part olive oil with one part acid—such as lemon juice, lime juice, balsamic vinegar, or apple cider vinegar—and some fresh or dried herbs. Add a little Dijon mustard or mayonnaise for flavouring. Or check your fridge for salad dressing—it makes a great marinade. For added flavour, sprinkle grilled vegetables with fresh herbs before serving.

Grilling and roasting times vary from veggie to veggie, but keep in mind that vegetables are generally more delicate than meats, so you'll need to keep a close eye on them to make sure they don't burn.

ROASTING VEGETABLES

Cut your vegetables into hearty bite-sized pieces and coat them with marinade. The longer they marinate, the more intense the flavour will be. Place the marinated veggies on a lightly greased baking sheet. Don't crowd them, or they will be more likely to steam than roast. Note that onions, mushrooms, and eggplant don't take as long to roast as carrots or potatoes, so either cut them into larger pieces or add them later.

Roast at 425°F, stirring every 10 to 15 minutes, for 45 minutes to an hour, or until the vegetables are tender, brown, and caramelized.

ROASTING GARLIC

While raw garlic is pungent, roasted garlic has a sweeter, milder flavour. To roast garlic, cut about ¼ inch off the pointed end of the garlic bulb. This will expose the tops of most of the garlic cloves in the bulb. Drizzle about ½ teaspoon of olive oil over the exposed cloves. Sprinkle the top with freshly ground sea salt and black pepper for more flavour.

Wrap a piece of tin foil around the garlic bulb and fold or twist the foil at the top to seal. Roast at 350°F for 30 or 40 minutes, or until the garlic cloves are golden brown and completely soft.

GRILLING VEGETABLES

Chop the vegetables into bite-sized pieces. The general rule is to cut the vegetables into pieces that will cook quickly and evenly. All pieces should be of consistent thickness and no more than about ¾-inch to 1-inch thick. Place the chopped veggies in a grilling basket or thread them on metal or bamboo skewers to keep them from falling into the fire. (If you're using bamboo skewers, soak them in water for 1 to 2 hours prior to using them to keep them from catching fire.)

Place the vegetables on the hot grill. If you are using skewers, turn after 5 to 7 minutes. If you have the vegetables in a basket, give the basket a shake after 5 to 7 minutes. If you're using a barbecue, keep the cover closed while cooking to capture some of that great smoky flavour. Most vegetables take about 5 to 10 minutes to cook, depending on the size and the vegetable. Do not overcook.

GRILLING FRUIT

While you have the grill going, you might as well grill your dessert too. When grilling fruit, you will want to choose one that is solid enough to hold together and maintain its texture on the grill. With many fruits, you can simply cut them in half. Split bananas lengthwise (leave the peel on to hold them together). Slice apples, pears, and similar fruits down the middle and remove the seeds and core. With most fruits, you can leave the peels on—whether you eat the skin or not. This helps to hold them together. Sliced pineapple is one of our favourite fruits to grill.

Before placing your fruit on the grill, ensure that the grate is very clean. If the fruit is small, use a grilling basket to prevent it from falling in the fire. Grill the fruit over medium direct heat until browned in spots and caramelized, turning once or twice. Cook for 8 to 10 minutes or until warm throughout.

Serve your grilled fruit with ice cream, yogurt, Nutella, or all the above. Top with ground cinnamon or nutmeg.

All about Legumes and Beans

Legumes are one of the most nutritious, versatile, and inexpensive foods available.

THE BENEFITS

Legumes such as chickpeas, kidney beans, black beans, navy beans, and lentils are simple foods with big benefits. They are chocked full of folate, vitamin B6, magnesium, potassium, zinc, and iron. They help regulate blood sugar, lower cholesterol and blood pressure, and guard against heart attack and cancer. Legumes are also an excellent source of fibre and vegetable protein, and they contain slowly absorbed carbohydrates.

Canada's Food Guide recommends that you get about three cups of beans per week to achieve the best health results. But even as little as a cup per week can help you achieve impressive results because beans and lentils offer protein, vitamins, minerals, and fibre with no added fat or cholesterol. Beans and lentils also count toward your daily vegetable servings to support good health. The fibre and protein in beans can help you feel satisfied, so you eat fewer calories overall. The lack of saturated fat in beans also makes them friendly to your waistline. One cup of beans or lentils contains between 200 and 230 calories.

USING CANNED LEGUMES

If you prefer the convenience of canned legumes, remember to drain them in a colander and rinse them under cool running water before adding them to your recipe. This removes excess sodium and many of the carbohydrates that produce intestinal gas.

STORING DRIED LEGUMES

Pour dried legumes into a clear vessel so you can easily see them. Store the jar or container in a cool, dry location, such as a cupboard or pantry. Keep the legumes away from direct sunlight to ensure they don't get rancid.

SOAKING DRIED BEANS

Dried lentils and split peas don't need to be soaked, but dried beans do. We prefer to use dried beans in the Eat Well kitchen. They cost less, have less additives and sodium, and taste better. There is also less waste from the cans.

Another benefit of soaking your dried beans is that this activates the germination process and reduces the problem of gas. Once wet, the beans release enzymes that begin to break down their gas- and indigestion-causing complex sugars into simple ones that are easier on your system. Soaking your beans overnight reduces sixty percent of the complex sugars in most beans.

Before soaking your beans, first inspect them for stones and then rinse them. Once this is finished, put them in a large bowl and fill it with three times more cold water than there are beans. Leave the beans to soak uncovered at room temperature (unless it is very warm because the beans might ferment). They should double in size after eight hours.

After the beans have soaked, rinse and drain them three or four times, or until the water runs clear.

COOKING REHYDRATED BEANS

After soaking and rinsing, place the rehydrated beans into a large pot and cover them with cold water. There should be at least an inch of water above the beans. Salt will prevent the beans from absorbing water, so don't add any salt until the beans are tender and cooked completely.

With the cover off, bring the water to a boil on high heat. Once boiling, a white foam will form on the surface from the gases being released from the beans. Skim the white foam off with a large spoon. Cover the pot, turn the heat down to low, and simmer gently.

Cooking times vary from bean to bean. The small-yet-mighty Adzuki bean takes 45 minutes to an hour to cook, while larger chickpeas or kidney beans can take up to an hour and a half to cook. As a rule of thumb, you should keep checking all beans every few minutes after 45 minutes of cooking time. Make sure that the beans are soft before you remove them from the heat—a hard bean can ruin an otherwise perfect meal.

In the Eat Well kitchen, we soak and cook a large pot of beans and then freeze the leftovers in zippered freezer bags. They can be defrosted in a bowl of warm water or added to a recipe while still frozen.

IDEAS FOR USING LEGUMES

Below are some tips to help you add legumes to your meals on a regular basis. We've also included several recipes for beans and lentils in this book.

- **Toss cooked legumes into leafy green and pasta salads.**

- **Add chickpeas to your favourite Greek salad recipe for a boost of protein and fibre.**

- **Make soup from dried beans or lentils or thicken soups and stews with pureed beans.**

- **Create a mixed-bean salad by combining red and white kidney beans with black beans. (The more types of beans, the prettier the salad.)**

- **Add cooked legumes to homemade or store-bought soups and stews.**

- **Make hummus and spread it on sandwiches.**

- **Add cooked chickpeas to grain dishes such as couscous or rice pilafs.**

- **Use half the amount of lean ground meat in tacos and burritos and make up the difference with beans.**

- **Add white kidney beans to a tomato-based pasta sauce for a Mediterranean-inspired meal.**

How to Make Milk or Soy Milk Yogurt

I make yogurt twice a week. Soy milk yogurt for my husband, Mike, and skim milk yogurt for me. I usually make two-litre batches because that is what my container holds, so you can double this recipe if you wish.

When you make yogurt, you are culturing good bacteria to make more good bacteria, and you want to make sure that all the bad bacteria is killed. To do this, you'll need to sterilize the container and lid that you're incubating the yogurt in.

You should begin by putting 2 to 3 tablespoons of existing plain yogurt starter (it should have live culture but no gelatin) into your sterilized jar, and then putting it aside to reach room temperature.

To make 1 litre of yogurt, place ⅓ cup of milk powder (or soy milk powder if you are making soy yogurt) in medium-sized saucepan. Whisk in 1 litre of milk. You can use skim milk, 2%, whole milk, or soy milk. (When using soy milk, I like the unsweetened variety of So Nice brand the best.)

Heat the milk on high for 5 minutes, whisking continually so it doesn't burn. Keep stirring and turn the heat down to medium. Continue until just before it comes to a boil or reaches 185°F. (Use a candy thermometer to check the temperature.)

Place the pot of milk in a larger pot containing cold water to cool it down. (If you do this in the sink, you will save a lot of mess.) You may want to change the water after about 5 minutes to keep it cold. Cool the milk mixture to 110°F.

Whisk the cooled milk into the container with the yogurt starter. Fasten the lid. Keep the yogurt warm and incubate by keeping the temperature as close to 100°F as possible. (Bacteria—good or bad—grows best at around 100°F.) Here are some options on keeping your milk at the correct temperature:

- **Use a yogurt maker**
- **Use a food dehydrator**
- **Use the pilot light in your oven**
- **Preheat oven to 100°F, or use the lowest temperature setting and then turn the oven off but leave the interior light on to maintain the temperature. You can check the oven temperature by putting a candy thermometer in a bowl of water in the oven.**

- **Wrap warm blanket(s) around your container**
- **Use a crock pot or slow cooker on its lowest setting or heated up then turned off**
- **Use a rice cooker's warm setting (i.e. plugged in, but with the cook function turned off)**

Leave the yogurt to incubate until it looks thick, usually any time after 5 to 7 hours. The longer you let it sit beyond 7 hours, the thicker and tangier it will become. Once the yogurt has finished incubating, store it in your refrigerator. It will keep for 1 to 2 weeks.

Whey, a thin yellow liquid, will form on the top of your yogurt when it's left sitting. You can pour the whey off or stir it in before eating your yogurt.

If you like a thicker yogurt, strain the yogurt through a cheesecloth. To do this, place the cheesecloth in a colander and then put the colander in a bowl large enough to catch the whey. Pour the yogurt in the colander, cover the colander with a plate, and put it all in the refrigerator. Strain for a couple of hours or overnight, depending on how thick you like it.

If you like your yogurt sweetened or with fruit, you can add your favourite sweetener or fruits anytime after it has incubated.

If you're planning on using some of your homemade yogurt as a starter for your next batch, use it within 7 days so that the bacteria still has growing power.

How to Thicken Sauces

Some people stay away from thickening sauces because they think it's difficult, but it is actually pretty easy. Keep reading to find out why and how.

HOW TO THICKEN A SAUCE USING ROUX

Roux, which is used to thicken sauces, is made from equal parts fat and flour. You can make a roux out of any fat, including the pan fat from roasted meat.

To make roux, place a skillet over medium-high heat and add your fat. Add an equal amount of flour and whisk or stir the mixture with a wooden spoon.

If you are making a white sauce such as béchamel, you'll only want to cook the roux for a few minutes so it doesn't brown. If you want to make a darker sauce, reduce the heat and cook the roux until it is the colour you wish. Be careful not to burn it.

Once your roux has reached the desired colour, slowly add your sauce liquid to the skillet while whisking or stirring. Let the mixture come to a boil and then turn the heat to low and let simmer, stirring often and skimming off any scum or fat that rises to the top. Most roux-thickened sauces need to be simmered for at least 20 minutes to cook out any starchy taste created by the flour.

HOW TO THICKEN A SAUCE USING CORNSTARCH SLURRY (GLUTEN-FREE OPTION)

If you wish to keep your sauce gluten-free, you can use a cornstarch slurry to thicken it instead of a flour-based roux. Cornstarch is also commonly used to thicken stir-fries and many Asian dishes.

To make a cornstarch slurry, dissolve your cornstarch with any cold liquid that is not acidic, like lemon juice is. One tablespoon of cornstarch will thicken two cups of liquid.

Bring your sauce liquid to a boil in a saucepan over medium-high heat. Whisk the slurry into the boiling sauce liquid and let it boil for 1 minute (cooking the sauce too long may cause it to thin). Remove the sauce from heat.

HOW TO THICKEN A SAUCE USING A VEGETABLE PURÉE

You can also use a cooked vegetable purée to thicken a sauce. For example, sautéed onions that have been braised with a pot roast can be strained out, puréed, and whisked back into the braising liquid to create a flavourful rustic sauce with no added fat.

Sometimes adding puréed vegetables and reducing is enough to thicken a sauce on its own, particularly with marinara sauce. Regardless, most sauces made from puréed vegetables benefit from some simmering and reducing, so I'd suggest trying this first before adding a roux or slurry. If you are planning on reducing your sauce, go easy on the seasonings so they won't be too strong.

You can also partially purée a soup to add some body to it by whizzing it with your hand blender when the soup is fully cooked. You can do this with any bean- or vegetable-based soup.

How to Prepare Eggplant for Cooking

Have I mentioned that I'm an eggplant enthusiast? I think I could write a whole cookbook about this delightful vegetable. And since I am such a fan, I'm going to refer to it by its more exotic French name: aubergine.

There are many wonderful dishes that include aubergine, such as caponata, eggplant parmesan, ratatouille, moussaka, and baba ghanouj. There are also several ways to prepare it. You can grill it, bread and fry it, stir-fry it, marinate it...the possibilities are endless!

The aubergine is a nightshade vegetable that contains nicotinoid alkaloids, which causes its slightly bitter taste. Salting the aubergine will pull out the juices that carry the bitter flavours. Salting also collapses the air pockets in the aubergine's sponge-like flesh, thus preventing it from absorbing too much oil and getting greasy.

When shopping for your aubergine, look for one with firm skin and no bruises. If the tip is brown and not a forest green, the inside will have already started to turn brown.

To salt your aubergine, slice, cube, or quarter it, depending on the recipe. Sprinkle the pieces generously with salt and let them sit in a colander for 30 minutes to an hour or two (you'll usually see a lot of liquid beading on the surface). Once they have finished sitting, rinse the aubergine pieces in water to remove the salt. Squeeze the aubergine a few pieces at a time in the palm of your hand to draw out the moisture, and then pat the pieces dry with paper towels. (Thorough drying is important—squeezing out excess moisture will give you a less oily result.)

When cooking the aubergine, you'll need to make sure it's completely done. It should be meltingly soft, smooth, and creamy—only then will it be flavourful on its own, as well as receptive to other flavours in your recipe.

The Mystery of Miso

Miso is a thick paste made from fermented soybeans and barley or rice malt. It is commonly used in Japanese cooking to make soups or sauces.

Most misos are made from soybeans, a grain, and sea salt. They can vary from dark and robust miso to mild red miso or sweet white miso.

From sweet, creamy, and light to hearty, robust, and dark, miso can be used to enhance everything from basic macrobiotic dishes to gourmet fare. The key to fine miso cookery is not to overpower dishes with a strong taste, but to integrate the more subtle aspects of miso's colour and flavour into a gentle balance with other ingredients. To realize the full potential of sweet miso, explore its uses in salad dressings and sauces. In contrast, dark, saltier misos combine nicely with beans, gravies, baked dishes, and vegetable stews and soups. Remember that dark misos are stronger in taste than sweet misos, so use them sparingly.

As a salting agent, miso supplies much in terms of flavour and nutrition without the harshness of salt. When substituting miso for salt, approximately 1 level tablespoon of a sweet, light miso or 2 level teaspoons of a dark, salty miso will take the place of ¼ teaspoon of salt.

Miso typically comes as a paste in a sealed container requiring refrigeration after opening. Natural miso is a living food containing many beneficial microorganisms that can be killed by overcooking. For this reason, I recommend that you add the miso to your dishes just before they are removed from the heat. Using miso without any cooking is even better.

How to Make Your Own Garam Masala

Garam masala is a pungent ground spice mixture often used in Northern Indian cuisine (and in the Eat Well kitchen!). It is available in many supermarkets and Indian grocery stores.

You can also use our recipe below to make a batch of your own garam masala. It can be made ahead and stored in an air-tight container for several months.

- **3 to 4 large cardamom pods, seeds only**
- **2 tbsp. cumin seeds**
- **2 tbsp. coriander seeds**
- **1 tbsp. black peppercorns**
- **1 (2-inch) cinnamon stick, broken up**
- **6 to 8 whole cloves**
- **½ tsp. grated fresh nutmeg**

1. Heat a dry skillet on medium to low heat. Add all of the ingredients and gently roast, stirring occasionally, for about 10 to 12 minutes, or until they turn several shades darker and give off a sweet smoky aroma.

2. Turn off the heat and allow the spices to cool. Once cooled, grind the spices to a fine powder in a clean, dry coffee grinder.

How to Make Great Risotto

You have got to love the Italians for coming up with the idea of risotto. Risotto is gluten-free, so it is easy on your tummy. The rice that is used in this dish absorbs the delicious flavours it is cooked in and then releases starches that make it creamy. If it is cooked properly, the risotto will be rich and creamy but still with some resistance or bite (al dente). If risotto is on the menu when I go to a restaurant, I'm ready to order!

Classic risotto is made from either carnaroli or arborio rice. Short and plump, these rices are high in starch and can absorb quite a bit of liquid without becoming mushy. Risotto can be made using many kinds of vegetables, meat, fish, seafood, or legumes. Different types of wine and cheese may also be used.

Cooking any type of risotto is based on a standard procedure. You'll use stock as your base of flavour. Your stock should complement the flavours of the risotto. For instance, use vegetable stock with the same seasonings or flavours as the recipe.

First, heat your stock in a saucepan, as a hot stock will cook into the risotto more quickly and evenly. While the stock is heating, sauté some onions or shallots in a large saucepan over medium heat in butter or olive oil. (They both add great flavour, but if you want to make your risotto dairy-free or vegan, use the olive oil.) This is the soffritto stage. After the onions or shallots have softened, add the rice and toast it in the pan. You'll know it's ready when the rice turns translucent at the edges. This is the tostatura stage.

If the recipe calls for wine, add it now to continue building the flavour. Continue cooking until the wine has evaporated, then raise the heat to medium-high and gradually add the hot stock 1 ladle at a time while stirring constantly but gently. Stirring loosens the starch molecules from the outside of the rice grains so they can melt into the surrounding liquid, creating a smooth, creamy texture.

Mantecatura is the last, essential step in making a risotto. To do this, remove the pan from heat and vigorously stir in butter, olive oil, or Parmesan cheese. (At the mantecatura stage, a vegetable purée may also be used as a low-fat alternative to butter.) This step binds the ingredients together, giving the risotto that characteristic and desirable creaminess.

It takes about 20 to 25 minutes to cook a risotto to al dente after the tostatura stage. Making risotto takes a little bit of practice to begin with, and a certain amount of concentration thereafter. Risotto is very sensitive to timing.

Properly cooked risotto is rich, velvety, and creamy but still with some resistance or bite. It should shimmer a little in the bowl and be fluid rather than a solid scoopful.

Whole Grains Cooking Chart

Grains (1 cup dry)	Water (cups)	Time (minutes)	Yield (cups)
Amaranth	2	25	2½
Barley, pearled	3	50–60	3½
Buckwheat groats*	2	15	2½
Cornmeal (polenta, coarse)	4–4½	20–25	2½
Couscous	2	instant	2½
Millet, hulled	3–4	20–25	3½
Oat groats	3	30–40	3½
Oat bran	2½	5	2
Quinoa	2	15–20	2–3
Rice, arborio	2	20	3
Rice, brown, basmati	2½	35–40	3
Rice, brown, long grain	2½	45–55	3
Rice, brown, short grain	2	45–55	3
Rice, brown, quick	1¼	10	2
Rice, wild	3	50–60	4
Rye, berries	3–4	60	3
Teff	3	5–20	3½
Wheat, bulgur	2	15	2½
Wheat, whole berries	3	120	2½

If you are cooking 1 cup of grains, use a 2-quart saucepan. Place the grains and water in your saucepan. Cover and bring to a boil over high heat. Reduce the heat down to low and steam for the recommended cooking time.

Lift the lid and test the grains for tenderness. If the grains need more time, cover the saucepan and steam 5 to 10 minutes longer.

When tender, turn off the heat and allow the grains to rest 5 to 10 minutes before fluffing and serving.

Buckwheat is the exception to the basic directions. Because the grain is so porous and absorbs water quickly, it's best to bring the water to a boil first before adding the buckwheat. When the water returns to a boil, cover the saucepan, turn the heat down to low, and time the steaming process.

Snacks and Apps

This chapter contains some interesting ideas for snacks and appetizers. Some are vegan and gluten-free, such as Theresa's Hummus *(page 30)* and Really Good Tapenade *(page 26)*. I've also included some recipes for those who like meat. If you wish to be the "belle of the ball," there are a couple of recipes that your friends or guests have probably never heard of, such as Bette Davis Eyes *(page 26)* and Dukkah *(page 28)*.

Karin's Crazy Cheese Ball

vegetarian
gluten-free

We served this on the cheese platters for catering functions, and it is very often requested when I am invited to a potluck.

- **2 cloves garlic, peeled**
- **I (250g) package cream cheese**
- **I cup shredded cheddar cheese**
- **½ cup crumbled blue cheese**
- **I tbsp. stone-ground Dijon mustard**
- **I tsp. cumin seeds, toasted**
- **I tsp. freshly ground pepper**
- **I tsp. Worcestershire sauce**
- **I tsp. dried dill**
- **I tsp. fresh parsley**
- **pinch cayenne pepper**
- **3 tbsp. chopped fresh parsley plus extra* for garnish**
- **toasted ground nuts* for garnish**

I. Place a piece of plastic wrap in the bottom of a small bowl and set aside.

2. In the food processor with the blade running, add the garlic cloves and process until well minced. Turn off food processor, open it, and add the remaining ingredients. Close the processor and process until well blended. Remove the contents with a rubber spatula and place onto the plastic in the bowl.

3. Put the bowl in the fridge and let the contents chill for an hour. Remove the bowl from the fridge and lift the mixture out of the bowl by picking up the four corners of the plastic. Remove the plastic wrap and mould the cheese mixture into a ball. Roll the cheese ball in your choice of chopped parsley, toasted chopped nuts, or a combination of both. Serve with vegetables or crackers. Makes about 2 cups.

*Optional

Here is a cheesy joke for you that my daughter Corinna told me because I can never pronounce Worcestershire correctly:

Jack and Joe were sitting at the table eating steaks. Each had a bottle of sauce for the steak. Joe wanted to try Jack's sauce and asked "Which is your sauce?"

Prosciutto, Cantaloupe, and Mozzarella Skewers

vegetarian
gluten-free

I found this recipe years ago and I've used it many times for various catering and family functions. These are always the first to go! I usually do a few without the prosciutto for the vegetarians.

- ½ cup (packed) fresh basil
- 1 medium shallot, quartered
- ½ cup olive oil
- 1 cantaloupe
- 20 thin slices of prosciutto (about ½ lb.)
- 20 water-packed mozzarella balls
- 20 (6-inch) wooden skewers

1. Make the dressing in a food processor by pulsing the basil and shallot together until minced and then slowly adding the olive oil thru the feed tube. Set aside. (This can be made ahead and stored in the refrigerator if you wish.)

2. Use a melon baller to get about 20 melon balls from the canteloupe. To get a perfect round melon ball, press the melon baller down firmly so it digs into the flesh, then twist to make the circle. I usually cut my melon in half and then scoop out the balls. That way, the juice stays inside.

3. Separate the prosciutto slices in a fan and set aside. Thread each of your wooden skewers with a mozzarella ball, then the prosciutto, and finally with a melon ball.

4. Arrange the skewers decoratively on a platter and drizzle the dressing over them just before serving. Makes 20 appetizers.

Sweet Potato and Goat Cheese Quesadilla Appetizers

vegetarian

This is an easy appetizer to prepare. You can make the filling the day before. You can also replace the goat cheese with feta, cheddar, or mozzarella and the cilantro with fresh dill, basil, or parsley. Serve with salsa and/or sour cream.

- **1 lb. sweet potatoes, peeled and diced**
- **2 tbsp. maple syrup**
- **¼ tsp. ground cinnamon**
- **1 tsp. vegetable oil**
- **½ cup chopped green onions**
- **2 cloves garlic, minced**
- **¼ cup chopped cilantro**
- **8 (6-inch) flour tortillas**
- **½ cup crumbled goat cheese**

1. Place the sweet potatoes in a medium saucepan filled with water over high heat. Bring to a boil and cook until the sweet potatoes are soft, about 15 to 20 minutes. Drain the potatoes and mash them with the maple syrup and cinnamon. Set aside.

2. Heat the oil in a skillet over medium-high heat. Add the onions and garlic and sauté for 1 to 2 minutes. Add the onion and garlic mixture and the cilantro to the sweet potato mixture, stirring until they are evenly combined.

3. Preheat the oven to 425°F. Lay four of the tortillas on a work surface. Divide the sweet potato mixture evenly among the tortillas and spread to the edges. Sprinkle each tortilla evenly with ⅛ cup goat cheese. Cover each of the filled tortillas with one of the remaining plain tortillas and press gently to stick.

4. Place the tortillas on a lightly greased baking sheet and bake for 7 to 10 minutes, or until browned. Remove from the oven and let them sit 3 to 4 minutes. Using a pizza slicer, cut each quesadilla into wedges and serve with salsa and/or sour cream. Serves 6 to 8.

Sweet potatoes are very nutritious. The most abundant vitamin found in a sweet potato is vitamin A. Each sweet potato gives you more than 300% of your recommended daily intake of vitamin A. Sweet potatoes also contain high levels of beta carotene and vitamins C, B5, and B6. One sweet potato contains about 112 calories.

Fresh Vietnamese Spring Rolls

vegan option
gluten-free

These soft, uncooked rolls served cold with a traditional dipping sauce make a refreshing change to deep-fried spring rolls. To make them, nutritious fillings—including noodles, shrimp, fresh vegetables, and aromatic herbs—are wrapped in delicate rice paper sheets. You can prepare these rolls up to 4 hours ahead and chill them in the refrigerator, covered with a clean dampened dish towel to keep them moist, until you're ready to serve. For a meatless option, replace the shrimp with tofu.

Vietnamese Spring Rolls

- ¼ (8 oz.) package rice vermicelli noodles
- 8 large cooked shrimp, peeled, deveined, and cut in half lengthwise
- 1½ tbsp. thinly sliced Thai basil
- 3 tbsp. chopped cilantro
- 2 large lettuce leaves, chopped
- ½ cup bean sprouts
- ½ cup peeled and grated carrot
- 1 tbsp. Bragg Liquid Aminos
- 2 tbsp. fresh lime juice
- 1 clove garlic, minced
- 1 tbsp. brown sugar
- 8 (8½-inch) rice wrappers

1. Fill a large saucepan with water and bring to a boil over high heat. Add the vermicelli and boil for 4 minutes. Drain and rinse the noodles in cold water.

2. Place the cooked vermicelli noodles in a large bowl and add the shrimp, Thai basil, cilantro, lettuce, bean sprouts, and carrot. In another small bowl, whisk together the Bragg's, lime juice, garlic, and sugar. Add the liquid mixture to the shrimp and vegetable mixture and stir to combine. Set aside.

3. Fill a large bowl with warm water. Dip a rice wrapper into the water for 1 second to soften. Lay the wrapper flat on a clean surface. Place 2 tablespoons of the filling mixture in a row across the centre of the wrapper, leaving about 2 inches uncovered on each side. Fold the uncovered sides inward and then close the wrapper by folding one of the large sides over the filling and rolling tightly. Repeat with the remaining wrappers and filling. Serve cold with traditional dipping sauce (recipe below). Makes 8 rolls.

Traditional Dipping Sauce

- 6 tbsp. ketchup
- 2 tsp. Worcestershire sauce
- 2 tsp. Bragg Liquid Aminos
- 2 tsp. sesame oil
- 1 tbsp. Asian chili sauce

1. Combine the ingredients in a small bowl and serve with spring rolls.

Bette Davis Eyes

vegetarian
gluten-free

I'm not the one that named this recipe—this came from a collection of recipes that I received from my friend Heather. Despite the strange name, these snacks are delicious and popular. They are also easy to prepare (but don't tell your friends) and can be made in advance.

- **8 oz. fresh white goat cheese (at room temperature)**
- **25 seedless red and/or green grapes**
- **1 cup pistachios, finely chopped**

1. Pack about 1 teaspoon of goat cheese around each grape and roll it in the palm of your hand until the cheese is smooth and the grape is evenly coated.

2. Place the chopped pistachios in a small bowl. Roll each grape in the nuts until it is evenly covered.

3. Cut each grape in half and arrange the halves on a serving tray. Makes 50 pieces.

Really Good Tapenade

vegan
gluten-free

You might be surprised to find out that tapenade gets its name not from the olives it contains but from capers, an essential ingredient in many tapenades. In the Occitan region in the south of France, the word for capers is "tapéno," hence the name for this popular spread. Tapenade can be served with vegetables, fish, or meat, and is sometimes used as a stuffing. It is often simply spread on artisan bread, pita, crostini, or crackers for use as an hors d'oeuvre. Some use it as a sandwich spread, while others use it to top baked potatoes or toss with pasta.

- **1 cup pitted mixed olives**
- **½ cup sun-dried tomatoes, sliced**
- **2 anchovies (optional)**
- **3 cloves garlic, minced**
- **2 tbsp. capers**
- **1 tsp. finely chopped fresh rosemary or thyme**
- **2 to 3 fresh basil leaves**
- **½ cup roughly chopped fresh parsley**
- **1 tbsp. freshly squeezed lemon juice**
- **2 tbsp. olive oil**

1. Rinse the olives thoroughly. Place all of the ingredients in the bowl of a food processor. Process to combine, stopping to scrape down the sides of the bowl, until the mixture becomes a coarse paste, approximately 1 to 2 minutes in total. Transfer the mixture to a bowl before serving. Makes 2 to 2½ cups.

Note: The tapenade will keep in a sealed container in the fridge for a couple of weeks in the unlikely event that you don't eat it all at once.

Baked Falafel Appetizers

vegan
gluten-free

This is a nice, easy appetizer to make. Serve these tasty falafels with our tahini sauce (page 70) and fresh veggies. You could even put some of our hummus (page 30) on the plate.

If you don't have a gluten restriction, you can also place the falafels in small pitas with sprouts, halved grape tomatoes, green onions, and tahini sauce.

- **3 cloves garlic, peeled**
- **4 green onions, sliced**
- **3 cups cooked chickpeas, rinsed and drained**
- **2 tbsp. olive oil**
- **2 tsp. ground cumin**
- **2 tsp. ground coriander**
- **2 tsp. sea salt**
- **1 tsp. paprika**
- **1 tsp. ground turmeric**
- **¼ tsp. cayenne pepper**
- **1 tsp. baking soda**
- **½ cup chopped fresh parsley**

1. Preheat the oven to 350°F.

2. Place the garlic in the bowl of a food processor and process until minced. Add the green onions and mince. Add the chickpeas and olive oil and blend until smooth but thick. Add the remaining ingredients and process until combined. The mixture should still be thick.

3. Drop the mixture onto a lightly greased baking sheet in tablespoon-sized dollops. Bake for 25 or 30 minutes, or until golden brown. Makes about 20 falafels.

Dukkah

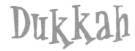

vegan
gluten-free

Dukkah is a unique and wonderful Egyptian spice and nut mix usually served with olive oil and crusty bread or pitas. You dip the bread in the olive oil and then the dukkah. The more you eat it, the more addictive it becomes.

If you have some leftover dukkah, it is one of the ingredients in the Persian Honey-Spiced Chicken recipe on page 154. Have that for dinner tomorrow!

- **1 cup whole hazelnuts**
- **½ cup sesame seeds**
- **2 tbsp. coriander seeds**
- **2 tbsp. cumin seeds**
- **1 tbsp. fennel seeds**
- **1 tbsp. black and/or pink peppercorns**
- **1 tsp. sea salt**

1. Preheat the oven to 350°F.

2. Place the hazelnuts on a baking sheet and bake for about 5 minutes, or until fragrant. While the nuts are still hot, pour them onto a tea towel. Fold the towel over them to cover, and then rub vigorously to remove the skins. Set the nuts aside to cool.

3. In a dry skillet over medium heat, toast the sesame seeds until light golden brown. Pour the seeds into a medium bowl as soon as they are done so they do not continue toasting.

4. In the same skillet, toast the coriander, cumin, and fennel seeds and the peppercorns while shaking the pan or stirring occasionally, cooking until the seeds begin to pop. Transfer the mixture to a food processor or spice grinder. Process until finely ground, and then pour into the bowl with the sesame seeds.

5. Place the cooled hazelnuts into the food processor and process until coarsely ground. Stir into the bowl with the spices.

6. Season the nut mixture with the sea salt and mix well. Makes about 2 cups.

This keeps well in a sealed jar for several weeks.

Holy Guacamole!

vegan
gluten-free

I like to make my guacamole chunkier like salsa rather than smooth, but you can do yours whichever way you choose. Either way, it's delicious served with corn chips or an array of fresh vegetables.

When choosing an avocado, check it for ripeness by gently pressing the outside. If there is no give, the avocado is not ripe yet and will not taste good. If there is a little give, the avocado is ripe. If there is a lot of give, the avocado may be past ripe and not good. In this case, taste test before using.

- **3 avocados, peeled and pitted (reserve one of the pits)**
- **1 lime, zest and juice**
- **½ tsp. salt**
- **½ cup diced red onion**
- **3 tbsp. chopped fresh cilantro**
- **2 plum tomatoes, diced**
- **2 garlic cloves, peeled and minced**
- **½ jalapeño pepper, minced (wear gloves)**
- **½ tsp. ground cumin**
- **½ tsp. freshly ground pepper**

1. Cut the avocados into chunks using a pastry blender or a knife and a fork and place them in a medium-sized bowl. Add the lime zest and juice and the salt. Mix in the onion, cilantro, tomatoes, garlic, and jalapeño pepper. Stir in the cumin and pepper.

2. Place the reserved avocado pit into the mixture. Cover the bowl with plastic wrap and refrigerate for 1 hour before serving. Makes 3 to 4 cups.

Theresa's Hummus

vegan
gluten-free

My sister Theresa and I used to make copious amounts of hummus and eat it all week. We called it birth control because of the vast amount of garlic we used. It's wonderful served with sliced veggies or pita bread.

If you rinse the cooked chickpeas with cold water, it reduces the extra gas that the beans may cause.

- **3 to 4 cloves garlic (less if you don't need birth control)**
- **2 cups cooked chickpeas, drained and rinsed**
- **3 to 5 tbsp. lemon juice**
- **2 tbsp. tahini**
- **¼ to ½ cup hot water**
- **½ tsp. sea salt**
- **½ tsp. cayenne pepper (if you want it spicy)**
- **2 tbsp. olive or sesame oil***

1. Place the garlic in a food processor and process until minced. Add the chickpeas, lemon juice, tahini, and ¼ cup of the water. Process until smooth, adding additional water until the mixture reaches the thickness you prefer.

2. Add the sea salt, cayenne, and olive or sesame oil. Blend for 3 to 5 minutes, or until thoroughly mixed and smooth. Makes about 2½ cups.

*Optional

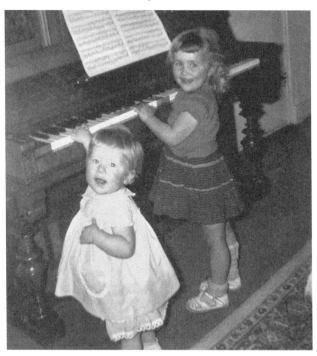

This picture is of my sister Theresa (right) and me.
Theresa was about four years old and I was two. Weren't we cute?

Skordalia

vegetarian
gluten-free option

Skordalia is a Greek garlic dip that can also be used as a spread or condiment. You can also make a gluten-free version with potatoes by substituting one boiled and mashed potato for the bread crumbs.

- **3 garlic cloves, peeled**
- **¼ tsp. sea salt**
- **1 cup chopped fresh parsley**
- **1 cup olive oil, divided**
- **1 lemon, zest and juice**
- **¼ cup dried bread crumbs**
- **½ cup crumbled feta cheese**
- **1 tbsp. dried oregano**
- **1 tbsp. capers, drained**
- **¼ tsp. freshly ground pepper**

1. Place the garlic in the bowl of a food processor and process until minced. Add the salt, parsley, ½ cup of the olive oil, and the lemon juice and process until combined. Add the remaining ½ cup of oil and the bread crumbs, feta cheese, oregano, capers, and pepper. Process for 1 minute and serve immediately or refrigerate. Makes about 2 cups.

Vegan Mushroom Pâté

vegan
gluten-free

My friend Sue has been after me to make this recipe for a long time. Both she and you will be pleased to see it in print.

Toasting the nuts for this dish either in the oven or in a dry skillet intensifies their flavours.

- **½ cup vegetable stock**
- **½ red onion, chopped**
- **4 cloves garlic, and minced**
- **2 cups any type of mushroom, roughly chopped**
- **2 tsp. dried sage**
- **2 tsp. dried rosemary**
- **½ tsp. ground nutmeg**
- **1 tsp. dried thyme**
- **2 tsp. Bragg Liquid Aminos**
- **½ tsp. sea salt**
- **1 tsp. freshly ground pepper**
- **2 tsp. balsamic vinegar**
- **1 tbsp. ground flaxseed**
- **1 cup walnuts, toasted**
- **½ cup roughly chopped fresh parsley**
- **parsley sprigs for garnish**

1. Pour the stock into a large saucepan over medium-high heat and bring to a boil. Add the onion, garlic, mushrooms, sage, rosemary, nutmeg, thyme, Bragg's, sea salt, and pepper and simmer for 10 to 15 minutes, or until the liquid has been absorbed and evaporated. Stir in the balsamic vinegar and ground flaxseed. Set aside.

2. Place the toasted walnuts and chopped parsley in the bowl of a food processor and pulse until combined. Add the mushroom mixture and pulse until smooth.

3. Scoop the pâté into a serving dish and garnish with parsley sprigs. Refrigerate for at least 2 hours before serving. Makes about 1½ cups.

Sunflower Herb Pâté

vegan

I saw this recipe in a magazine, but changed it around a bit to suit my taste. I used to sell wedges of this at the local farmers' market. This is delicious on a sandwich or bagel with maple mustard or served on crackers.

- 1½ cups unsalted sunflower seeds, toasted and divided
- 2 unpeeled potatoes, washed and grated
- ¼ cup spelt flour
- 2 tbsp. extra virgin olive oil
- 3 tbsp. nutritional yeast
- ½ onion, roughly chopped
- 2 tbsp. lemon juice
- 2 tsp. dried basil
- 2 tsp. dried sage
- 2 tsp. dried oregano
- 2 tsp. dried dill
- 1 tsp. sea salt
- 3 cloves garlic, minced
- 1 tbsp. Bragg Liquid Aminos
- 1 tsp. or more freshly ground pepper

1. Preheat the oven to 350°F.

2. Place all ingredients except ½ cup of the sunflower seeds into a food processor and blend until they reach a uniform consistency. Adjust the seasoning to taste.

3. Spoon the mixture into a lightly greased pie pan and smooth out as best you can. Sprinkle the mixture with the remaining ½ cup of sunflower seeds. Bake for 30 to 35 minutes, or until firm. Cool and cut into wedges before serving. Makes 8 wedges.

Curry and Walnut-Stuffed Mushrooms

vegan
gluten-free

Stuffed mushrooms are awesome! They are easy to make, great for parties, and the variations are endless. You can get as creative as you like with the filling. This stuffed mushroom recipe is perfect for anyone on a gluten-free or vegan diet. But if your guests don't have restrictions, top these with some grated Parmesan cheese.

- **20 to 24 white button mushrooms**
- **3 tbsp. olive oil, divided**
- **2 small shallots, minced**
- **2 cloves garlic, minced**
- **3 tbsp. chopped walnuts**
- **1 apple, peeled, cored, and diced**
- **½ tsp. sea salt**
- **½ tsp. freshly ground pepper**
- **2 tbsp. chopped fresh parsley**
- **2 tsp. curry powder**
- **2 tbsp. sherry or vegetable stock**

1. Preheat the oven to 375°F.

2. Wipe the mushrooms with a paper towel. Remove the stems and chop them coarsely. Set the caps aside.

3. Heat 1 tablespoon of the olive oil in a small skillet over medium-high heat. Add the chopped mushroom stems and shallots and sauté for 4 to 5 minutes, stirring often. Add the garlic, walnuts, and apple and then sprinkle with the salt. Stir well and sauté for 2 more minutes.

4. Stir in the pepper, parsley, curry powder, and the sherry or stock. Sauté and stir for 1 more minute and remove the skillet from the heat.

5. Toss the mixture into a food processor and pulse several times until it gets crumbly. Set aside.

6. Toss the mushroom caps with the remaining 2 tablespoons of olive oil. Fill each mushroom with the stuffing and place on a baking pan. Bake for 20 to 25 minutes. Allow to cool for 5 minutes before serving. Makes about 24 appetizers.

Note: Once they are cooked, stuffed mushrooms do not hold up well for long periods. Try baking them in smaller batches, serving, and repeating.

So Awesome Sicilian Caponata

vegan
gluten-free

You've got to hand it to the Sicilians for coming up with this terrific and tasty combination of vegetables and flavours. It can be spooned onto some good crusty bread or used as a topping on grilled chicken. It also goes great with pasta. The possibilities are endless!

- **¼ cup pine nuts, toasted**
- **1 large eggplant, cubed and salted***
- **3 or more tbsp. olive oil, divided**
- **1 red onion, diced**
- **2 stalks celery, diced**
- **2 cloves garlic, minced**
- **1 green bell pepper, diced**
- **3 Italian tomatoes, diced**
- **1 tsp. sea salt**
- **¼ cup Thompson raisins**
- **¼ cup pitted Sicilian green olives, quartered**
- **¼ cup red wine vinegar**
- **2 tbsp. capers, drained**
- **1 tbsp. sugar**
- **½ tsp. freshly ground pepper**
- **2 tbsp. chopped fresh basil**

1. In a small, dry skillet, cook the pine nuts over medium heat, stirring often until lightly toasted. Set aside.

2. Rinse the salted eggplant pieces, drain them, and pat them dry with a clean tea towel or paper towel.

3. In a large skillet, heat 1 tablespoon of the olive oil over medium-high heat. Add the eggplant in batches and sauté (using more oil if needed) until golden brown. Transfer to a bowl and set aside.

4. In the same skillet, heat 1 tablespoon of the remaining oil over medium heat. Add the onion, celery, and garlic and sauté until softened, about 4 to 5 minutes. Add the green pepper, tomatoes, and sea salt. Cook and stir for 5 minutes, or until the pepper has softened. Stir in the raisins, olives, vinegar, capers, sugar, and pepper. Return the eggplant to the pan and stir in the last tablespoon of oil.

5. Cover the skillet and simmer for 10 to 15 minutes. Remove from heat and allow the mixture to cool for 10 minutes. Stir in the pine nuts and basil immediately before serving. Makes about 5 to 6 cups.

*For detailed instructions on salting eggplants, see page 17.

Note: You can refrigerate this caponata in an airtight container for up to 1 week. Let it come to room temperature before serving.

Mango Tango Salsa

vegan
gluten-free

Fresh mango salsa is easy to make and perfect as an appetizer served with corn chips or as a main alongside any type of grilled fish. Frozen mango works just as well as fresh in this recipe, but be sure to thaw it first.

If you would like more heat in your salsa, add the other half of the jalapeño pepper before serving.

- **2 cloves garlic, peeled**
- **1 (thumb-sized) piece fresh unpeeled ginger, chopped**
- **½ jalapeño pepper, chopped (use gloves)**
- **2 cups peeled and roughly chopped mango**
- **1 red bell pepper, roughly chopped**
- **1 green bell pepper, roughly chopped**
- **½ cup roughly chopped red onion**
- **1 lime, zest and juice**
- **½ cup chopped fresh cilantro**
- **sea salt to taste**
- **freshly ground pepper to taste**

1. Place the garlic, ginger, and jalapeño in the bowl of your food processor and pulse until minced. Add the mango, red and green peppers, and onion. Pulse off and on until the fruit and vegetable pieces have been chopped to the size of corn kernels.

2. Move the ingredients into large bowl and mix well. Add the lime zest and juice and the cilantro. Season with salt and pepper. Cover and chill. This can be made up to 6 hours ahead of time. Makes 4 to 5 cups.

Soup's On!

This chapter contains some of our more popular soup recipes. We served soup at the Charlottetown Farmers' Market every Saturday. Many of our regular clients will be excited to see the recipes for African Chickpea and Peanut Stew *(page 38)*, Cuban Black Bean Soup *(page 39)*, or Sam's favourite, Fresh Garden Gazpacho *(page 41)*.

Moroccan Red Lentil Soup

vegan
gluten-free

I'm in love with the fragrant combination of seasonings that the Moroccans use. The warmth of the turmeric and cumin combined with the pungent flavour of the saffron makes an excellent combination.

Red lentils are great for soup. They are small, so they cook faster than brown or green lentils. After cooking they soften and tend to purée easily. For a smoother texture to this soup, you can purée it with a hand blender.

- 1 tbsp. sunflower or olive oil
- 2 onions, chopped
- 4 cloves garlic, minced
- 1 tbsp. grated unpeeled fresh ginger*
- 2 stalks celery, chopped
- 1½ tsp. sea salt
- 1 tsp. freshly ground pepper
- 1 tsp. ground turmeric
- 1 tsp. ground cumin
- 1 tsp. ground cinnamon or 1 (6-inch) cinnamon stick
- pinch saffron
- 6 cups water or vegetable stock
- 1 cup red lentils
- 1 tbsp. tomato paste
- 2 unpeeled potatoes, washed and cubed
- 1 (796 ml) can diced tomatoes
- 1 cup frozen peas
- 2 tbsp. chopped fresh parsley
- vegan sour cream (page 67) for garnish

1. Heat the oil in a large soup pot or Dutch oven over medium-high heat. Add the onions, garlic, ginger, and celery, stirring occasionally until softened, about 5 minutes. Add the sea salt, pepper, turmeric, cumin, cinnamon (if using ground cinnamon), and saffron. Cook, stirring often, for 2 minutes.

2. Add the water or stock, lentils, tomato paste, potatoes, tomatoes, and cinnamon stick (if not using ground cinnamon) and bring to boil. Reduce heat, cover, and simmer for 35 minutes.

3. Add the peas and simmer until the lentils, vegetables, and potatoes are tender, about 10 more minutes. Add the parsley and remove from heat. If desired, serve with a dollop of sour cream. Serves 8.

* Unless your ginger has a thick tough peel, it is fine to grate the peel with the rest of the ginger.

African Chickpea and Peanut Stew

vegan
gluten-free

This was the most popular soup that we served at the local farmers' market. It's perfect for cold weather, loaded with protein, and vegan and gluten-free!

- 1 tbsp. sunflower oil
- 1 large onion, chopped
- 1 red bell pepper, diced
- 1 green bell pepper, diced
- 2 garlic cloves, minced
- 1 tbsp. ground coriander
- 1 tbsp. ground cumin
- 1 tsp. cayenne pepper
- 1½ tsp. dried parsley or
  3 tbsp. chopped fresh parsley
- 1 cup uncooked brown rice
- 8 cups vegetable stock
- 1 (6-inch) cinnamon stick
- ⅔ cup crunchy peanut butter
- 2 large sweet potatoes, peeled and diced
- 2 cups cooked chickpeas, rinsed and drained
- crushed peanuts for garnish

1. Heat the oil over medium heat in a large soup pot. Add the onion and sauté until soft, about 3 to 4 minutes. Add the red and green peppers and the garlic and cook, stirring occasionally, for about 5 minutes, or until the peppers are soft. Turn up the heat to high and add the coriander, cumin, cayenne, parsley (if using dried), and rice. Keep stirring until it is very hot and aromatic, about 3 to 5 minutes.

2. Add the stock and cinnamon stick and bring to a boil. Turn the heat to low and simmer, covered, for 40 minutes, stirring occasionally.

3. Add the peanut butter, sweet potatoes, and chickpeas one at a time, stirring well between additions. Bring the mixture to a boil over high heat. Reduce the heat to low, cover, and simmer for 5 to 10 minutes, or until the rice and sweet potatoes are tender.

4. Serve in bowls garnished with crushed peanuts and fresh parsley (if not using dried). Serves 8 to 10.

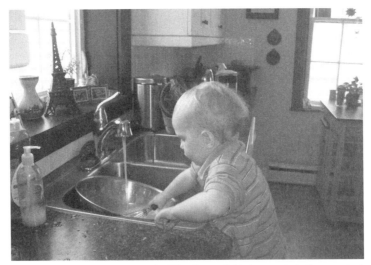

This is my grandson Piercen. He is also goes by "The Peanut." He loves to help Grammy in the kitchen!

Cuban Black Bean Soup

vegan
gluten-free

This is Eric McEwen's favourite soup and Eric MacEwen is one of my favourite people. (Eric is a well-known broadcaster of East Coast Music and hosts a weekly show syndicated around the Maritimes. He is also a founding director of the East Coast Music Awards.)

The small size of the black beans in this dish isn't indicative of their nutritional content. In fact, black beans are rich in folate, magnesium, phosphorus, and iron. They're also high in fibre and vegetarian protein and low in fat. What's more, black beans contain virtually no artery-clogging saturated fat.

- **2 tbsp. sunflower oil**
- **2 onions, diced**
- **4 stalks celery, chopped**
- **4 carrots, peeled and sliced**
- **1 green bell pepper, diced**
- **4 cloves garlic, minced**
- **1½ tsp. ground cumin**
- **2 tsp. dried oregano**
- **1 chipotle or jalapeño pepper, minced (wear gloves)**
- **½ tsp. sea salt**
- **½ tsp. freshly ground pepper**
- **3 cups cooked black beans, rinsed and drained**
- **1 (798 ml) can diced tomatoes**
- **6 cups vegetable stock**
- **2 bay leaves**
- **½ cup chopped fresh cilantro**

1. Heat the oil in a soup pot over medium heat. Add the onions and sauté for 2 to 3 minutes. Add the celery, carrots, green pepper, and garlic and sauté for another 3 to 4 minutes. Add the cumin, oregano, chipotle or jalapeño pepper, sea salt, and pepper and cook for another minute.

2. Stir in the black beans, diced tomatoes, vegetable stock, and bay leaves. Bring to a boil, and then reduce the heat to low and simmer, covered, for an hour.

3. Once the soup has finished simmering, remove the bay leaves and discard them. Then use a hand blender to purée the soup until it is at the thickness you desire. Stir in the cilantro before serving. Serves 6 to 8.

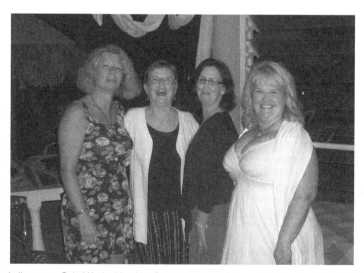

Martini Monday ladies go to Cuba! Karin, Heather, Sue, and Lori in Cuba celebrating Sue's 50th birthday April 2012

Low-Fat Leek and Potato Soup

vegan
gluten-free

We try to keep our soups vegan and gluten-free to allow more options for people on specialized diets. This version of leek and potato soup does just that.

- **2 tbsp. sunflower or olive oil**
- **3 medium leeks (the white and green parts), washed well and sliced thin**
- **1 large onion, coarsely chopped**
- **3 cloves garlic, minced**
- **3 carrots, peeled and chopped**
- **4 stalks celery, sliced**
- **1 tbsp. dried dill**
- **½ tsp. grated fresh nutmeg**
- **1 tsp. sea salt**
- **½ tsp. freshly ground pepper**
- **1 tbsp. Bragg Liquid Aminos**
- **3 to 4 large unpeeled potatoes, washed and cubed**
- **5 cups vegetable stock**
- **1½ cups unsweetened soy milk or milk**
- **3 tbsp. chopped fresh parsley**

1. Place the oil in a large soup pot and heat over medium-high heat. Add the leeks and onion and sauté for 3 to 4 minutes. Add the garlic, carrots, and celery and sauté for another 3 to 4 minutes.

2. Stir in the dill, nutmeg, sea salt, pepper, and Bragg's. Next add the potatoes and vegetable stock and stir to combine.

3. Bring the mixture to a boil, cover, and let simmer 30 to 35 minutes, or until the potatoes and carrots are tender. Once the soup has finished simmering, remove it from the heat and add the soy milk or milk.

4. Purée the soup with a hand blender until the soup is uniformly smooth. Before serving, reheat the soup, adjust the seasonings to taste, and add the fresh parsley. Serves 6 to 8.

Fresh Garden Gazpacho

vegan
gluten-free

This is an excellent chilled soup to make during the height of summer when all these vegetables and herbs are bursting with flavour and colour. This recipe is for you, Sailboat Sam!

- **3 lbs. fresh garden tomatoes**
- **1 yellow pepper**
- **1 large fennel bulb**
- **½ red onion**
- **3 stalks celery with leaves**
- **2 tbsp. chopped fresh parsley**
- **4 cloves garlic, minced**
- **1 tbsp. olive oil**
- **2 tbsp. red wine vinegar**
- **1 tsp. Bragg Liquid Aminos**
- **1 tsp. freshly ground pepper**
- **pinch cayenne pepper**
- **3 cups cold vegetable stock**
- **1 bunch fresh basil, sliced thinly**

1. Chop all of the vegetables, the parsley, and the garlic or pulse them in the food processor until they are about the size of corn kernels. Place the mixture in a large bowl. Add the olive oil, red wine vinegar, Bragg's, black pepper, cayenne pepper, and vegetable stock and mix well.

2. Season to taste and garnish with basil. Serve chilled. Serves 4 to 6.

Basic Miso Soup

vegan
gluten-free

Miso soup is a staple of Japanese cuisine. For my husband Mike and me, it is one of the more comforting foods. It is good for your tummy, has a light and mild flavour, and is quick and easy to prepare. For more information about miso, check out page 18.

- **3 cups water**
- **1 tbsp. shredded nori or wakame seaweed***
- **½ pound firm tofu, cut into 1-inch cubes**
- **3 green onions, chopped**
- **¼ cup miso**
- **½ tsp. Bragg Liquid Aminos****
- **½ tsp. sesame oil****

1. Bring the water to a boil over high heat in a medium-sized saucepan. Reduce the heat to low and add the seaweed, tofu, and green onions. Allow to simmer at least 5 to 6 minutes.

2. Reduce the heat to very low and add the miso. Stir until the miso is well dissolved. It is best not to boil the miso, as this will ruin some of its healthy properties as well as change the flavour of the soup.

3. Season to taste with Bragg's and sesame oil. Serves 3 to 4.

* Nori is a seaweed that comes in sheets. It is often used in rolling sushi. Wakame is a sea vegetable or edible seaweed. It has a subtly sweet flavour and is most often served in soups and salads.

**Optional

Spicy Asian Noodle Soup

vegan
gluten-free

Here is a good, healthy soup for clearing the sinuses. Reduce the amount of chili sauce used if you wish for a less exciting flavour.

- 1 tbsp. sunflower oil
- 2 onions, diced
- 2 scrubbed or peeled carrots, sliced on the bias
- 2 stalks celery, sliced on the bias
- 1 stalk lemongrass
- 2 tbsp. grated fresh unpeeled ginger
- 4 cloves garlic, minced
- 8 cups vegetable stock
- 2 tbsp. Bragg Liquid Aminos
- 1 tbsp. Asian chili sauce
- 1 cup soy beans, cooked and rinsed, or 1 cup firm tofu, cubed
- ½ (454 g) package rice vermicelli
- 1 tbsp. shredded nori seaweed
- 3 green onions, chopped
- 1 tbsp. chopped fresh cilantro
- ¼ cup miso
- 1 tbsp. sesame oil

1. Heat the oil in a large pot over medium-high heat. Add the onions, carrots, and celery and sauté for 4 to 5 minutes.

2. Remove the tough outer leaves of the lemongrass and cut off the bulb, about an inch from the end. Slice the remaining tender parts into thin slices and add to the pot along with the ginger and garlic. Sauté for another 1 to 2 minutes.

3. Add the vegetable stock, Bragg's, chili sauce, and soy beans or tofu and bring to a boil. Let simmer over low heat for 15 to 20 minutes.

4. Add the ½ package of noodles, breaking the noodles up a bit as you put them in the pot. Let simmer for another 3 minutes. When the mixture has finished simmering, turn off the heat and mix in the remaining ingredients. Adjust the seasonings to your taste before serving if desired. Serves 8 to 10.

Good and Hearty Lentil Soup

vegan
gluten-free

This soup is chock-full of veggies and very yummy. Serve it with our Cornmeal Muffins from page 182.

- **1 tbsp. sunflower oil**
- **1 onion, chopped**
- **2 unpeeled carrots, scrubbed and diced**
- **2 stalks celery, chopped**
- **2 cloves garlic, minced**
- **1 tsp. dried oregano**
- **1 tsp. dried basil**
- **2 cups uncooked green and/or brown lentils**
- **1 (796 ml) can crushed tomatoes**
- **8 cups water**
- **2 bay leaves**
- **2 cups fresh spinach, rinsed and thinly sliced, or 1 (10 oz.) package frozen**
- **2 tbsp. vinegar**
- **sea salt to taste**
- **freshly ground pepper to taste**

1. In a large soup pot, heat the oil over medium heat. Add the onion, carrots, and celery. Cook and stir for 2 to 3 minutes, or until the onion is tender. Stir in the garlic, oregano, and basil and sauté for 2 minutes. Add the lentils, tomatoes, water, and bay leaves and bring the mixture to a boil. Reduce the heat to low and simmer, covered, for at least 1 hour, or until the lentils are tender.

2. When ready to serve, stir in the spinach and cook until it wilts or melts. Add the vinegar and season to taste with salt and pepper and more vinegar if desired. Serves 8 to 10.

Roasted Parsnip Soup

vegan
gluten-free

Even those who aren't fans of parsnips enjoy this soup. Roasting the vegetables enhances their natural sweetness.

- **3 lbs. parsnips, peeled and cut into 1-inch pieces**
- **3 carrots, scrubbed, peeled, and cut into 1-inch pieces**
- **1 large onion, diced**
- **4 cloves garlic, peeled**
- **2 tbsp. olive oil, divided**
- **1 tsp. Bragg Liquid Aminos**
- **½ tsp. freshly ground pepper**
- **3 stalks celery, diced**
- **1 tsp. unpeeled fresh ginger, grated**
- **1 tbsp. brown sugar**
- **½ tsp. ground cardamom**
- **½ tsp. ground allspice**
- **½ tsp. ground nutmeg**
- **¼ tsp. cayenne pepper**
- **6 cups vegetable stock**
- **2 tbsp. chopped fresh parsley**

1. Preheat the oven to 425°F.

2. Place the parsnips, carrots, onion, and garlic into a large bowl. Sprinkle the vegetables with 1 tablespoon of the olive oil, the Bragg's, and the freshly ground pepper. Toss to coat.

3. Spread the vegetables evenly over a baking sheet. Roast in the preheated oven for about 30 minutes, or until the parsnips are tender and golden brown. Set aside.

4. Heat the remaining tablespoon of oil in a large soup pot over medium heat. Stir in the celery and ginger and cook for 2 to 3 minutes. Turn up the heat to high and stir in the brown sugar, cardamom, allspice, nutmeg, cayenne, and the roasted vegetables, reserving ¼ cup of the roasted parsnips.

5. Pour in the vegetable stock and bring to a boil. Reduce the heat to low and simmer, covered, until all of the vegetables are very tender, about 15 to 20 minutes.

6. Remove the soup from heat and whiz with a hand blender until it is puréed. Chop the reserved roasted parsnips and stir them into the soup. Garnish with the parsley. Serves 6 to 8.

Creamy Sun-Dried Tomato and Chickpea Soup

vegan
gluten-free

Tahini is the secret ingredient that makes this delicious soup so nice and creamy. Tahini is a ground sesame paste that is a source of the healthy fatty acids omega-3 and omega-6. It can be purchased in any Middle Eastern grocery store.

- 1 tbsp. sunflower oil
- 1 medium onion, chopped
- 2 to 3 cloves garlic, minced
- 1 large unpeeled carrot, scrubbed and sliced
- 2 cups cooked chickpeas, drained and rinsed
- 1 (796 ml) can crushed tomatoes
- 5 to 6 sun-dried tomatoes, chopped
- 1 tsp. ground cumin
- ¼ tsp. freshly ground pepper
- pinch cayenne pepper
- ½ tbsp. apple cider vinegar
- 1 tbsp. Bragg Liquid Aminos
- 2 cups vegetable stock
- 2 tbsp. tahini
- 2 tbsp. chopped fresh parsley

1. Heat the oil in a large soup pot over medium-high heat. Add the onion, garlic, and carrot and sauté for 2 to 3 minutes, or until the onion is soft.

2. Add the chickpeas, crushed tomatoes, sun-dried tomatoes, cumin, pepper, cayenne, vinegar, Bragg's, and vegetable stock. Bring to a boil, then reduce heat and simmer covered for 20 minutes, or until the carrots are tender.

3. Remove the pot from the heat and stir in the tahini. Purée the soup with a hand blender until smooth. Garnish with the fresh parsley before serving. Serves 4 to 6.

Salivating Salads

Salads don't just have to be a mix of greens (although a mix of greens can be very tasty). Our salads have a variety of ingredients, such as beans, rice, grains, or potatoes. Some of our clients' salad faves include Greek Pasta Salad *(page 48)*, Mediterranean Couscous Salad, *(page 49)* and Chillin' Chickpea and Artichoke Salad *(page 54)*.

Curried Rice Salad
with Apples and Chickpeas

vegetarian
vegan option
gluten-free

This salad is healthy, it has lots of flavour, and it's a great way to use up leftover rice. Bring it to your next potluck!

- **2 cups cooked brown rice**
- **5 green onions, sliced**
- **2 stalks celery, chopped**
- **1 medium unpeeled apple, cored and chopped**
- **½ cup raisins**
- **1 red bell pepper, diced**
- **1 cup cooked chickpeas, rinsed and drained**
- **¼ cup chopped fresh cilantro**
- **1 tsp. ground turmeric**
- **1 tsp. curry powder**
- **½ tsp. sea salt**
- **2 tbsp. regular or soy yogurt**
- **2 tsp. Worcestershire sauce**
- **1 tbsp. apple cider vinegar**
- **¼ cup lemon juice**
- **¼ cup olive oil**
- **freshly ground pepper to taste**

1. Mix the cooked rice, green onions, celery, apple, raisins, red pepper, chickpeas, and cilantro in a large bowl.

2. In a separate small bowl, whisk together the turmeric, curry powder, sea salt, yogurt, Worcestershire sauce, apple cider vinegar, lemon juice, and olive oil. Add the pepper and adjust the seasonings to your taste.

3. Pour the liquid mixture over the rice mixture and mix well to combine.

4. Serve at room temperature. Serves 4 to 6.

Turmeric grows wild in the forests of south and southeast Asia. It is one of the key ingredients in many Indian, Persian, and Thai dishes such as curry. Turmeric is currently being investigated for possible benefits in Alzheimer Disease, cancer, arthritis, and other clinical disorders. I love it for the earthy flavour and the beautiful color.

Greek Pasta Salad

vegetarian

This salad is loaded with vegetables, texture, and flavour. It was extremely popular with our clients. You know who you are!

- **½ cup olive oil**
- **1½ tsp. dried oregano**
- **½ cup red wine vinegar**
- **1 tsp. Dijon mustard**
- **freshly ground pepper to taste**
- **1 (450 g) package uncooked fusilli pasta**
- **1 red onion, thinly sliced**
- **½ cup black kalamata olives**
- **1 green bell pepper, diced**
- **1 red bell pepper, diced**
- **2 large tomatoes, diced**
- **1 cucumber, sliced**
- **1 cup crumbled feta cheese**
- **sea salt to taste**

1. Pour the olive oil, oregano, vinegar, Dijon, and black pepper in a jar with a tightly fitting lid. Close the lid and shake to combine. Set aside.

2. Cook the fusilli noodles according to directions on the package. Drain the noodles but don't rinse them. Place the fusilli in a large bowl.

3. Re-shake the olive oil mixture and pour half of the dressing over the hot pasta. Toss to mix well. Add the onion, olives, green and red peppers, tomatoes, and cucumber to the pasta and combine well. Add the feta cheese, reserving 2 tablespoons.

4. Pour the remaining dressing over the salad and toss well. Check your seasonings and adjust to your taste if necessary. Garnish with the reserved feta. Serves 4 to 6.

Mediterranean Couscous Salad

vegetarian

This salad is best served just after it is made. The ingredients can be prepared in advance, but the salad should be assembled at the last minute.

- **2 cups water**
- **2 cups uncooked instant couscous**
- **1 English cucumber, finely cubed**
- **½ cup chopped sun-dried tomatoes**
- **1 cup crumbled feta cheese**
- **3 tbsp. toasted pine nuts**
- **½ cup chopped fresh parsley**
- **1 lemon, zest and juice**
- **½ cup extra virgin olive oil**
- **sea salt to taste**
- **freshly ground pepper to taste**

1. Bring the water to a boil in a saucepan. Stir in the couscous, cover, and set aside for 10 minutes.

2. Once the couscous has finished resting, pour it into a large serving bowl. Break up the clumps using a fork or your fingers. Add the cucumber, sun-dried tomatoes, feta cheese, pine nuts, and parsley and toss.

3. In a separate small bowl, whisk the lemon zest and juice together with the olive oil. Pour the liquid over the salad. Season to taste with sea salt and pepper before serving. Serves 4 to 6.

Haida's Tabouli Salad

vegan
gluten-free

This is my daughter Haida's recipe. She serves it at room temperature or even slightly warm. I believe it is more flavourful that way. Serve it alone or with our Mjadra (page 116) and/or Baked Lebanese-Spiced Kibbee (page 168).

- **½ cup bulgur (cracked wheat)**
- **2 cups boiling water**
- **2 tomatoes, diced**
- **3 green onions, finely chopped**
- **1 large bunch fresh parsley, finely minced**
- **1 lemon, zest and juice**
- **3 cloves garlic, minced**
- **¼ cup olive oil**
- **1 tbsp. dried mint or 2 tbsp. fresh mint**
- **sea salt to taste**
- **freshly ground pepper to taste**
- **1 cup cooked chickpeas**

1. Put the bulgur in medium-sized bowl and cover it with boiling water. Set aside and let soak for 20 minutes.

2. In a separate large bowl, toss the tomatoes, green onions, and parsley together. Add the lemon zest and juice, garlic, olive oil, mint, salt, and pepper and mix to combine.

3. Drain the excess water from the bulgur and toss into the bowl with the vegetables. Add the chickpeas and mix well with your hands or large spoon. Serves 4.

The Wondrous Wheat Berry Salad

vegan

Wheat berries are delicious, great in salads, and give your jaws a good workout. The term "wheat berry" refers to the entire wheat kernel except for the hull, comprising the bran, germ, and endosperm.

- **1 cup hard winter wheat berries**
- **3 cups cold water**
- **3 green onions (white and green parts), sliced small**
- **½ green bell pepper, diced**
- **½ red bell pepper, diced**
- **1 unpeeled carrot, scrubbed and diced small**
- **1 cup cooked corn kernels, frozen or fresh**
- **4 tbsp. olive oil**
- **2 tbsp. orange juice concentrate**
- **2 tbsp. balsamic vinegar**
- **1 tbsp. maple syrup**
- **1 tsp. chopped fresh rosemary**
- **½ tsp. sea salt**
- **½ tsp. freshly ground pepper**

1. Soak the wheat berries for a couple of hours or overnight.

2. Drain the wheat berries, rinse them, and place them in a saucepan. Pour the cold water over the top. Cover and cook the wheat berries over low heat for approximately 45 minutes, or until they are soft. Drain.

3. In a large bowl, combine the warm wheat berries with the green onions, red and green peppers, carrot, and corn.

4. In a separate small bowl, whisk together the olive oil, orange juice concentrate, balsamic vinegar, maple syrup, rosemary, salt, and pepper. Pour over the salad and toss. Allow the salad to sit for at least 30 minutes for the wheat berries to absorb the sauce.

5. Season to taste and serve at room temperature. Serves 4.

Roasted Corn, Pepper, and Jicama Salad

vegan
gluten-free

Jicama (pronounced HEE-kah-mah) is also known as the Mexican potato. It is a root vegetable with a unique sweet flavour and the texture of a radish. It goes well in salads, salsas, and vegetable platters.

- **2 medium ears of corn**
- **1 medium jicama, peeled and cut into thin strips**
- **1 medium red onion, thinly sliced**
- **1 small red bell pepper, cut into thin strips**
- **1 small green bell pepper, cut into thin strips**
- **1 small jalapeño pepper, seeded and minced (wear gloves)**
- **2 tbsp. red wine vinegar**
- **2 tbsp. extra virgin olive oil**
- **2 tbsp. water**
- **½ tsp. dry mustard**
- **½ tsp. sea salt**
- **1 clove garlic, minced**
- **freshly ground pepper to taste**

1. Preheat the oven to 400°F.

2. Place the ears of corn on a baking sheet and roast corn 25 to 30 minutes, or until tender. Let the corn cool, and then remove the kernels from the cobs.

3. Placing the corn kernels into a large salad bowl. Add the jicama, onion, bell peppers, and jalapeño and toss to combine.

4. In a separate small bowl, whisk together the vinegar, olive oil, water, mustard, salt, garlic, and pepper. Add to the vegetables and toss to coat. Serves 4 to 6.

Quinoa and Sweet Potato Maple Salad

vegan
gluten-free

This salad is high in protein and flavour, but low in fat. Whole grain quinoa cooks quicker than most grains and is an excellent source of protein—there are 11 grams of protein per cup of cooked quinoa! Serve this salad slightly warm or at room temperature.

- **½ cup uncooked quinoa**
- **1 cup vegetable stock or water**
- **1 small sweet potato, peeled, boiled, and diced**
- **2 cups fresh spinach**
- **1 red bell pepper, diced**
- **3 tbsp. lemon juice**
- **2 tbsp. olive oil**
- **1 tbsp. maple syrup**
- **2 tsp. Dijon mustard**
- **1 tbsp. chopped fresh rosemary or basil or ½ tsp. dried rosemary or basil**
- **sea salt**
- **freshly ground pepper**

1. Rinse the quinoa in a sieve under cold water for 2 to 3 minutes while stirring with your hand.

2. After rinsing, toast the quinoa in a dry saucepan over high heat, stirring constantly for 2 to 3 minutes. Add the stock or water and bring to a boil. Cover, reduce the heat to low, and simmer for 15 to 20 minutes, or until the water has been absorbed and the quinoa is light and fluffy. Remove from heat and allow to cool.

3. In a large bowl, toss together the quinoa, sweet potato, spinach, and red pepper.

4. In a separate small bowl, whisk together the lemon juice, olive oil, maple syrup, Dijon mustard, and rosemary or basil. Gently fold the dressing into the quinoa mixture. Season with sea salt and pepper to taste before serving. Serves 4.

Scrumptious Sushi Rice Salad

vegan
gluten-free

With this salad, you get all the delicious flavours of sushi without the extra work of rolling.

- 1½ cups uncooked short-grain sushi rice
- 1¾ cups plus 2 tbsp. water, divided
- ¼ cup seasoned rice vinegar
- 1 tbsp. sugar
- 1 tsp. salt
- 1¼ tsp. wasabi paste
- 1 tbsp. sesame oil
- 1 medium carrot, peeled and cut into ½-inch slices
- 1 red bell pepper, cut into ½-inch slices
- 3 green onions, thinly sliced diagonally
- 3 tbsp. drained and sliced Japanese pickled ginger, coarsely chopped
- 1 ripe avocado
- 1 tbsp. toasted sesame seeds
- 2 sheets toasted nori, cut into 1-inch strips with scissors

1. In a medium-sized bowl, rinse the rice in several changes of cold water until the water is almost clear. Place the rice and 1¾ cups of the water in a large heavy saucepan and bring to a boil. Cover the saucepan and simmer on low heat for 2 minutes. Remove the saucepan from heat and let the rice stand, covered, for 10 minutes (do not lift the lid during this time).

2. While rice is standing, bring the vinegar, sugar, and salt to a boil in a small saucepan, stirring constantly. Cook until the sugar has dissolved. Set aside to cool.

3. When the rice has finished standing, place it in a large bowl. Sprinkle the rice with the vinegar mixture and toss to coat.

4. In a separate small bowl, whisk together the wasabi, the remaining 2 tablespoons of water, and the sesame oil. Add the dressing to the rice mixture and toss to coat. Add the carrot, red pepper, green onions, pickled ginger, and nori and toss gently.

5. Halve, pit, and peel the avocado. Cut it crosswise into ¼-inch slices. Arrange the avocado slices on top of the salad, then sprinkle the salad with the sesame seeds. Serves 4 to 6.

Chillin' Chickpea and Artichoke Salad

vegan
gluten-free

Once you chow down on some of this salad, you will be chilled out. I'm always looking for ways to include my favourite legume—the chickpea—in meals, and this is an excellent way. Sautéing the onion and garlic adds a nice sweetness to the salad. Serve this salad at room temperature.

- 1 tbsp. olive oil
- ½ red onion, diced
- ½ red bell pepper, diced
- 2 large cloves garlic, minced
- 1 tbsp. fresh rosemary or ½ tsp. dried rosemary
- 2 cups cooked chickpeas, rinsed and drained
- ¾ cup marinated artichokes plus 2 tbsp. of the marinade juice
- 1 lemon, zest and juice
- 2 tbsp. olive oil
- sea salt to taste
- freshly ground pepper to taste
- ½ cup chopped fresh parsley

1. Heat the 1 tablespoon of oil in a skillet over medium heat. Add the onion and sauté for 2 to 3 minutes. Add the red pepper, garlic, and rosemary and sauté for 2 to 3 minutes, or until soft. Set aside.

2. In a large bowl, combine the chickpeas and artichokes. Set aside.

3. In a separate small bowl, whisk together the artichoke juice, lemon zest and juice, 2 tablespoons of olive oil, sea salt, and pepper. Pour the mixture over the chickpeas and artichokes. Add the contents of the skillet. Mix well to combine all of the ingredients, and season to taste.

4. Let the salad stand for about 1 hour before serving. Serves 4.

Sesame Noodle Salad with Tahini Sauce

vegan
gluten-free

You can use any type of noodle for this salad. We chose rice noodles to keep it gluten-free.

You can buy black sesame seeds at any Asian grocery store. Mix them with some white sesame seeds and toast them for an attractive garnish.

- **1 (454 g) package rice vermicelli noodles**
- **1 green bell pepper, sliced**
- **1 red bell pepper, sliced**
- **1 large unpeeled carrot, scrubbed and grated**
- **2 garlic cloves, peeled**
- **½ cup well-stirred tahini**
- **¼ cup fresh lemon juice**
- **¼ cup water**
- **1 tbsp. Bragg Liquid Aminos**
- **¼ tsp. cayenne pepper**
- **3 tbsp. toasted sesame seeds**

1. Bring a large pot of water to a boil over high heat. Break up the rice noodles and add them to the water. Boil for 4 minutes, then drain and rinse well with cold water.

2. Place the noodles in a large salad bowl. Add the sliced green and red peppers and the grated carrot. Set aside.

3. Place the garlic in the bowl of a food processor and process until minced. Add the tahini, lemon juice, water, Bragg's, and cayenne and process until combined well.

4. Pour the tahini sauce over the salad and toss to combine. Sprinkle the salad with the toasted sesame seeds and serve. Serves 4 to 6.

Mediterranean Potato Salad

vegan
gluten-free

This is a lovely potato salad recipe that doesn't use mayonnaise, making it free of animal products.

Potato peels contain a lot of nutrients, so we keep them on for this recipe. Red and/or yellow potatoes are very nice for this salad.

- **2 lbs. unpeeled potatoes, washed and cubed**
- **2 cloves garlic, minced**
- **2 tbsp. olive oil**
- **3 tbsp. red wine vinegar**
- **1 tsp. Dijon mustard**
- **1 tsp. Bragg Liquid Aminos**
- **2 tsp. dried basil**
- **½ red onion, chopped**
- **2 red, yellow, or orange bell peppers (your choice), diced**
- **1 green bell pepper, diced**
- **2 tbsp. fresh chives**
- **½ tsp. sea salt**
- **freshly ground pepper to taste**

1. Place the potatoes in a large pot and cover with water. Bring to a boil over high heat. Reduce the heat to medium-low and cook for 15 to 20 minutes, or until tender. Drain well. Place the potatoes in a large bowl and set aside.

2. In a separate small bowl, add the garlic, olive oil, vinegar, Dijon, Bragg's, and basil and stir well to combine.

3. Pour half the dressing mixture onto the hot potatoes and gently stir, taking care not to break up the potato pieces too much. Add the remaining ingredients and toss to combine, adding more dressing if needed. Season to taste. Serves 4 to 6.

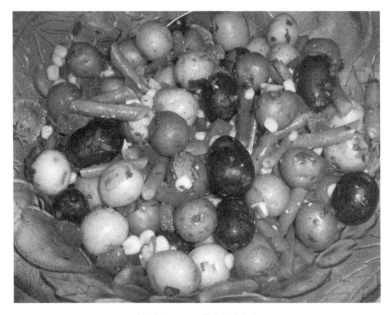

Mediterranean Potato Salad

On the Side

Here are some ideas to serve on the side with your main course of chicken, beef, or tofu. The Savoury Wild Rice, Cranberry, and Almond Pilaf *(page 64)* goes very well with the Herb-Roasted Chicken and Vegetables *(page 143)* and the Holiday Heaven Tofu *(page 92)*. And Mike's Favourite Sweet Potato Cakes *(page 62)* might just win over the heart of someone in your life.

Potatoes Anna Karin-ina

vegetarian (with vegan option)
gluten-free

I often serve these potatoes with my meat and chicken courses. For this dish, I changed the classic "Potatoes Anna" recipe by adding a few extra ingredients, so I chose to change the name also.

- **6 tbsp. butter***
- **2 cloves garlic, finely minced**
- **1 tsp. dried rosemary or 1 tbsp. fresh rosemary**
- **1 cup finely chopped green onions**
- **4 medium unpeeled Yukon Gold or Russet potatoes, washed and sliced very thin****
- **1 large unpeeled sweet potato, washed and sliced very thin****
- **sea salt to taste**
- **freshly ground pepper to taste**

1. Preheat the oven to 425°F.

2. Place the butter, garlic, and rosemary in a small saucepan over medium-low heat, and cook until the butter has melted.

3. Generously brush the bottom and sides of a 9-inch heavy ovenproof skillet with some of the butter mix. Arrange about half of the white potato slices in a single layer over the bottom of the skillet, overlapping them slightly. Brush the potato layer with some of the butter mixture, then sprinkle with one quarter of the green onions and season with sea salt and pepper.

4. Arrange half of the sweet potatoes over the first layer, and then brush them with butter and sprinkle another one quarter of the green onions and salt and pepper over them. Keep repeating these steps to add layers, alternating between the regular potatoes and the sweet potatoes, until all of the ingredients have been used.

5. When all of the layers are complete, place the skillet on the stove over high heat for 3 to 4 minutes. Remove the skillet from heat and cover it with some greased foil. Press down on the potatoes firmly to tamp them down.

6. Bake in the preheated oven for 30 minutes. Remove the foil and bake another 30 to 40 minutes, or until the potatoes are tender and golden. Remove from the oven and let cool for 5 minutes. Run a small spatula around the edges of the potatoes, and then slide a large spatula underneath to loosen them. Carefully invert the potatoes onto a cake plate. Cut the potato cake into 8 wedges and serve. Serves 6 to 8.

*For vegan option, use olive oil instead of butter.

**Do not place the potato slices in water before using because the starch is needed for binding.

Bubble and Squeak

vegetarian
gluten-free

How can you resist anything that has a name like Bubble and Squeak? This is a tasty potato and cabbage side dish that you can serve with any meat or tofu. It is an excellent way to use up any type of leftover potatoes. You can also add some turkey bacon to it for extra flavour. Any type of cabbage is fine to use, but I prefer Savoy.

- ½ **medium head cabbage, sliced**
- **I cup water**
- **2 tbsp. butter**
- **I onion, thinly sliced**
- **3 cups leftover cooked potatoes**
- ½ **tsp. paprika**
- **sea salt to taste**
- **freshly ground pepper to taste**

1. Place the cabbage and the water in a large skillet over medium-high heat and cook for about 5 minutes, or until tender. Drain and set aside.

2. Melt the butter over medium heat in another large skillet. Add the onion and sauté for 2 to 3 minutes, or until soft. Add the cooked potatoes and the cabbage and press down on the mixture with a spatula to form a cake. Fry, without stirring, until browned on the bottom. Flip the potato cake over and cook until the other side has also browned. Season with the paprika, sea salt, and pepper. Cut into wedges before serving. Serves 4.

Cumin Rice Pilaf

vegan
gluten-free

This tasty pilaf goes great with any curry dish or even on its own with some sautéed tofu and vegetables.

- **I tbsp. cumin seeds**
- **I large bunch green onions, thinly sliced**
- **I tsp. sunflower oil**
- **I½ cups uncooked white rice**
- **2 cups vegetable stock**
- **¾ cups water**
- **I tsp. Bragg Liquid Aminos**
- **freshly ground pepper to taste**
- ½ **cup finely chopped fresh parsley or cilantro**

1. In a medium saucepan over medium heat, sauté the cumin seeds and green onions in the oil until the onions have softened, about 1 to 2 minutes. Add the rice and cook, stirring frequently, for 1 minute. Stir in the stock, water, Bragg's, and pepper and bring to a boil over high heat. Cover the pan, reduce the heat to low, and cook until the liquid is absorbed and the rice is tender, about 15 minutes.

2. Remove the pan from heat and let stand, covered, for 5 minutes. Fluff the rice with a fork and toss with the parsley or cilantro before serving. Serves 4.

Turnip Puff

vegetarian

My husband, Mike, isn't a big fan of turnips, but he does love these turnip puffs. They are a regular at Christmas dinner. You can also substitute the turnip with cooked squash, sweet potato, or a combination of both.

- **4 cups peeled and diced turnip**
- **4 tbsp. butter, divided**
- **2 eggs, beaten**
- **3 tbsp. unbleached white flour**
- **1 tbsp. brown sugar**
- **1 tsp. baking powder**
- **½ tsp. freshly ground pepper**
- **½ tsp. sea salt**
- **pinch ground nutmeg**
- **¾ cup bread crumbs, cornflake crumbs, or nutritional yeast**
- **paprika to taste**

1. Preheat the oven to 375°F.

2. Place the turnip in a large saucepan and cover with water. Bring to a boil over medium-high heat and cook for 25 to 30 minutes, or until the turnip is tender. Drain the turnip, and then remove to a large bowl and mash.

3. Add 2 tablespoons of the butter and the eggs to the turnip and mix well. Next add the flour, brown sugar, baking powder, pepper, sea salt, and nutmeg and mix well to combine. Set aside.

4. Melt the remaining 2 tablespoons of butter and place in a separate small bowl. Add the bread crumbs and mix well.

5. Pour the turnip mixture into a lightly greased casserole dish. Spread the bread crumb mixture over the top, then sprinkle with paprika to taste. Bake in the preheated oven for 25 minutes, or until light brown on top. Serves 4 to 6.

Zucchini and Potato Pancakes with Sour Cream Caper Sauce

vegetarian

These pancakes are terrific during harvest season when zucchinis are plentiful. They go well alongside any main course or even on their own as the main course.

Zucchini and Potato Pancakes

- **2 large unpeeled potatoes, washed and grated***
- **2 medium unpeeled zucchinis, washed and grated**
- **2 cloves garlic, minced**
- **½ cup chopped green onion**
- **½ cup chopped fresh parsley**
- **4 eggs**
- **3 tsp. unbleached white flour**
- **½ tsp. sea salt**
- **½ tsp. freshly ground pepper**
- **1 to 2 tbsp. sunflower oil**

1. Preheat the oven to 250°F.

2. Place the potatoes, zucchini, garlic, green onion, parsley, eggs, flour, salt, and pepper in a large bowl and toss with your hands to combine. Be careful not to overmix.

3. Heat 1 tablespoon of the oil in a large skillet over medium-high heat. Cook the pancakes in batches by dropping large tablespoons of the potato mixture into the skillet and frying both sides until golden. Use more oil if needed.

4. Transfer the cooked pancakes to paper-towel-lined plates to drain. Keep them warm in the oven until ready to serve. Serve with Sour Cream Caper Sauce (recipe below). Serves 4 to 6.

Sour Cream Caper Sauce

- **½ cup reduced-fat sour cream or yogurt**
- **1 tbsp. capers, rinsed and chopped**
- **1 tsp. lemon juice**
- **½ tsp. dried dill**

1. Place all ingredients in a small bowl and stir well to combine.

*If you want to prepare the potatoes in advance, submerge them in a bowl of cold water immediately after grating them. When you're ready to cook, drain them well, then spread them on a clean cloth towel, roll it up, and squeeze it gently to remove the moisture.

Mike's Favourite Sweet Potato Cakes

vegan
gluten-free

This is another one of my husband Mike's faves. These cakes are nice warm or cold, served with a protein and a salad.

- **1 cup uncooked millet**
- **2 cups water**
- **2 sweet potatoes, peeled and cut into 2-inch cubes**
- **1 tbsp. sunflower oil**
- **1 onion, diced**
- **1 green bell pepper, diced**
- **1 red bell pepper, diced**
- **3 cloves garlic, minced**
- **1 tsp. dried basil**
- **1 tsp. dried parsley**
- **sea salt to taste**
- **freshly ground pepper to taste**
- **½ cup tahini**
- **1 tbsp. Bragg Liquid Aminos**
- **2 tbsp. toasted sesame seeds (a mix of white and black if you have them)**

1. Rinse the millet well in a sieve. Place it in a small pot over high heat and stir constantly until the millet starts popping, making sure it doesn't burn. Add the water and bring to boil. Cover, reduce the heat to low, and let simmer for 25 minutes, or until all the liquid has been absorbed.

2. While the millet is cooking, boil the sweet potatoes in a large covered saucepan over medium-high heat for 20 minutes, or until soft. Drain the potatoes, then replace them in the pan and mash well. Set aside.

3. Preheat the oven to 325°F.

4. Heat the oil over medium heat in large skillet. Add the onion and sauté for 3 to 4 minutes, or until translucent. Next add the green and red peppers and garlic and continue sautéing for another 3 to 4 minutes, or until soft. Mix in the basil, parsley, salt, and pepper. Remove the skillet from the heat and add the mashed sweet potatoes, cooked millet, tahini, and Bragg's. Stir to combine well.

5. Drop ½ cup-sized scoops of the mixture onto a lightly greased baking sheet about 1½ inches apart. Flatten each scoop slightly with a fork and shape into a cake. Garnish the cakes with the sesame seeds.

6. Bake in the top half of the oven for 45 minutes, or until firm. Makes about 12 cakes.

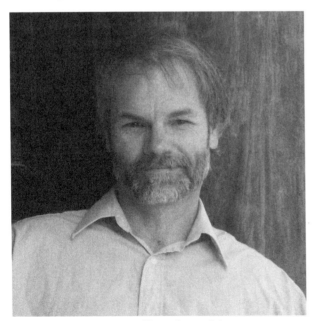

Mike, lover of Sweet Potato Cakes

Oven Potato or Sweet Potato Fries

vegan
gluten-free

These potato or sweet potato fries are delicious with the spice mixture recommended below, but you can also experiment with the flavour by using 1 to 2 tablespoons of chipotle powder, smoked paprika, Chinese five spice, garam masala, Cajun seasoning, or another spice of your choice. Or try making up your own spice combination—the possibilities are endless!

- **3 large unpeeled baking potatoes or sweet potatoes (or a mix of the two), washed and cut into uniform wedges**
- **2 tbsp. olive oil**
- **1 tsp. paprika**
- **1 tsp. granulated garlic powder**
- **1 tsp. chili powder**
- **1 tsp. onion powder**
- **1 tsp. dried oregano**

1. Preheat the oven to 450°F.

2. Place the potato wedges in a bowl and cover with very hot water. Let soak for 5 minutes.

3. While the potatoes are soaking, mix the olive oil, paprika, garlic powder, chili powder, onion powder, and oregano together.

4. Drain the potatoes and dry them with a clean tea towel. Once dry, place the potatoes back into the bowl and add the olive oil mixture. Toss well to coat the potatoes evenly.

5. Place on an ungreased baking sheet. Bake, stirring occasionally, for 35 to 45 minutes*, or until golden brown. Serves 4.

*Note that sweet potatoes cook faster than white potatoes, so make sure you check these often while cooking so they don't burn. If you are using a mix of sweet potatoes and regular potatoes, add the sweet potatoes 10 minutes after the regular potatoes.

Savoury Wild Rice, Cranberry, and Almond Pilaf

vegan
gluten-free

I serve this with Herb-Roasted Chicken and Vegetables (page 143) or Holiday Heaven Tofu (page 92). The wild rice adds a lovely texture to the pilaf.

- 1 tbsp. sunflower oil
- 1 onion, diced
- 1 unpeeled carrot, scrubbed and grated
- 3 cloves garlic, minced
- 1 cup uncooked organic brown rice
- 1 cup uncooked wild rice
- 1 tsp. dried parsley
- 1 tsp. dried sage
- ½ tsp. dried rosemary
- ½ tsp. dried thyme
- ½ tsp. freshly ground pepper
- 4 cups vegetable stock
- 1 tsp. Bragg Liquid Aminos
- ½ cup dried cranberries
- 3 tbsp. chopped fresh parsley
- ¼ cup slivered almonds, toasted*

1. Heat the oil in a large heavy skillet over medium-high heat. Add the onion, carrot, and garlic and sauté for 3 to 4 minutes, stirring often. Mix in the brown and wild rice, dried parsley, dried sage, dried rosemary, dried thyme, pepper, stock, Bragg's, and cranberries. Turn up the heat to high, cover, and bring to a boil. Reduce the heat to low and simmer for 40 to 45 minutes, or until the rice is tender.

2. Mix in the fresh parsley and adjust the seasonings to taste. Garnish with the toasted slivered almonds just before serving. Serves 4.

*To toast the nuts, spread them out in a single layer on a baking sheet. Bake in a 350°F oven, stirring occasionally, for 10 to 15 minutes. Or, toast the nuts in an ungreased skillet over medium heat, stirring for 5 to 10 minutes, or until golden brown and aromatic.

Vegetable Croquettes

vegetarian

These croquettes are healthy because they are full of vegetables and they are baked instead of fried. Serve them as a side with mustard or ketchup.

- **1 tbsp. sunflower oil**
- **2 tbsp. onion, minced**
- **2 cloves garlic, minced**
- **1 red bell pepper, diced**
- **2 cups grated carrot**
- **2 cups diced zucchini**
- **2 tomatoes, peeled and diced**
- **1 bay leaf**
- **½ tsp. dried oregano**
- **3 tbsp. butter**
- **¼ cup unbleached flour**
- **1 cup vegetable stock**
- **½ cup milk**
- **2 large eggs, beaten**
- **1 cup cooked brown or white rice**
- **¼ cup chopped fresh parsley**
- **1 tsp. grated lemon zest**
- **2 cups seasoned bread crumbs, divided**

1. Preheat the oven to 350°F.

2. Heat the oil in a large skillet over medium-high heat. Add the onion, garlic, and red pepper and sauté for 2 to 4 minutes, or until soft. Add the carrot, zucchini, and tomatoes and cook for 15 to 20 minutes, or until the vegetables are soft and the liquid has evaporated. Stir in the bay leaf and oregano. Remove from heat and set aside.

3. Melt the butter in a medium saucepan over medium heat. Add the flour and stir until it is well mixed. Turn the heat up to medium-high and slowly add the stock and the milk, stirring constantly. Keep stirring until the mixture comes to a boil. Reduce the heat to medium and stir for 3 or 4 minutes, or until thick. Beat in the eggs one at a time and continue to whisk until the mixture is well thickened, taking care not to let it boil.

4. Add the sauce, cooked rice, parsley, lemon zest, and 1½ cups of the bread crumbs to the sautéed vegetables. Mix well and let cool.

5. Coat your hands in flour and use your palms to roll the cooled mixture into 16 small balls. Shape the balls into cones and roll each cone in the remaining ½ cup of bread crumbs until evenly coated. Place the cones on a lightly greased baking sheet and bake for 45 minutes, or until lightly browned. Makes 16 croquettes.

into the Sauces and Dressings

Sauces can make a meal or salad. This chapter gives you the much sought-after recipe for our Eat Well Tomato Sauce *(page 67)*, which is used as a base for our lasagnas, barbecue sauce, Perfect Pizza Rustica *(page 169)*, and Scoobi Doo Pasta with Meat Sauce and Cheese *(page 170)*. There are also two recipes for the famous béchamel sauce, a regular version and a gluten-free version.

Eat Well Tomato Sauce

vegan
gluten-free

Here it is: the recipe everyone is always asking me for! This is the base recipe we used in the Eat Well kitchen for our lasagnas, pizzas, pasta dishes, etc. This recipe makes a large batch, so you can freeze some in individual containers and have it handy when you need it.

- **2 (798 ml) cans diced tomatoes, divided**
- **5 cloves garlic, sliced**
- **½ cup brown sugar**
- **½ cup balsamic vinegar**
- **2 tbsp. dried basil**
- **2 tbsp. dried parsley**
- **2 tbsp. dried oregano**
- **1 tsp. cayenne pepper**
- **2 (798 ml) cans crushed tomatoes**

1. Drain about 2 tbsp. of juice from the diced tomatoes and heat this in a large pot over medium heat. Add the sliced garlic and stir. Continue to cook for 5 to 7 minutes, or until soft, adding more juice by the tablespoon if it evaporates.

2. Mix in the remainder of the can of diced tomatoes, along with the brown sugar, balsamic vinegar, basil, parsley, oregano, and cayenne pepper. Bring the mixture to a boil and stir constantly for 4 to 5 minutes.

3. Add the remaining cans of diced and crushed tomatoes and bring to a boil. Reduce the heat to low and simmer, covered, for 45 minutes. Adjust the seasonings to taste. Makes about 14 cups.

Vegan Sour Cream

vegan
gluten-free

Sour cream is one of the things I pined for during the years I was a vegan. This is a very good substitute.

- **½ (12.3 oz.) package light silken tofu**
- **2 tbsp. chopped fresh cilantro**
- **1 tbsp. olive oil**
- **4 tsp. lemon juice**
- **2 tsp. apple cider vinegar**
- **1 tsp. honey**
- **½ tsp. sea salt**

1. Place all the ingredients in the bowl of a food processor and blend until very creamy and smooth. Makes about 1 cup.

Do the Salsa!

vegan
gluten-free

This homemade tomato salsa is especially good to make during the harvest season, when the veggies and tomatoes are ripe, plentiful, and sweet.

There is a lot of chopping involved in this recipe, but I happen to know that if you play some good Cuban music and practise salsa dancing while you're chopping, your recipe will turn out even better. Try it!

- **5 large Roma/plum tomatoes**
- **1 green bell pepper, diced**
- **4 stalks celery, chopped**
- **1 onion, chopped**
- **1 jalapeño pepper, seeded and minced (wear gloves)**
- **4 cloves garlic, minced**
- **1 lime, zest and juice**
- **2 tbsp. tomato paste**
- **1 tsp. sea salt**
- **1 tbsp. chopped fresh oregano or 2 tsp. dried oregano**
- **1 tsp. freshly ground pepper**
- **3 tbsp. chopped fresh cilantro**

1. Combine all of the ingredients except the cilantro in a large pot. If you would like fresh salsa to eat right away, remove as much as you'd like and refrigerate it. It will stay good for up to a week.

2. Bring the remaining vegetables to a boil over medium-high heat. Reduce the heat to medium. Cover and simmer, stirring often, for 10 minutes. Mix in the cilantro.

3. Remove the pot from heat and ladle the salsa into hot, sterilized jars. If the salsa is to be stored for a while, seal the jars and process them in a boiling water bath for 10 minutes before storing. (If you do not process the salsa jars in the boiling water bath, the salsa must be eaten within a week.) Makes about 6 cups.

Béchamel Sauce

vegetarian

Known as one of the "mother" sauces in classic French cuisine, béchamel is versatile: it's used in dishes such as lasagna, macaroni and cheese, and moussaka, and it can also serve as the base for soufflés, soups, and savoury pie fillings. For a gluten-free version of this sauce, see page 70.

To be able to say that I know how to make the famous béchamel sauce makes me feel like an accomplished chef. Don't tell anyone, but it's almost easier to make this sauce than it is to pronounce its name!

- **2 tbsp. butter**
- **2 tbsp. unbleached white flour**
- **2 cups milk**
- **½ tsp. grated fresh nutmeg**
- **sea salt to taste**
- **white pepper* to taste**

1. In a small saucepan, melt the butter over medium-low heat. Remove the pan from the heat, add the flour, and stir it into the butter to form a thick and smooth paste.

2. Pour in ½ cup of the milk and whisk until the mixture has transformed into a smooth white liquid with no lumps. Add the remainder of the milk and whisk.

3. Place the saucepan back onto the stove and turn the heat up to medium-high. Bring the liquid to a boil, stirring continuously. Once the sauce starts to boil and thicken, reduce the heat to low. Simmer for 5 to 10 minutes, stirring frequently, until thickened. Season with the nutmeg, sea salt, and pepper. Makes about 2 cups.

*White pepper is ideal for this recipe because the sauce is white and won't show the specks, but freshly ground black pepper is also fine.

Gluten-Free Béchamel Sauce

vegetarian
gluten-free

- **3 tbsp. cornstarch**
- **2 cups plus 4 tbsp. low-fat milk, divided**
- **½ tsp. grated fresh nutmeg**
- **sea salt to taste**
- **white pepper* to taste**

1. Place the cornstarch in a small bowl and mix in 4 tablespoons of the milk, stirring until smooth. Set aside.

2. Pour the remaining 2 cups of milk and the nutmeg in a large saucepan over medium-high heat. Stir constantly until it comes to a boil.

3. Re-stir the cornstarch mixture and slowly add it to the boiling milk, stirring constantly. Keep stirring until the sauce comes to a boil again and reduces to the consistency of very thick cream, about 2 minutes. Remove from heat and season to taste with salt and pepper. Makes about 2 cups.

*White pepper is ideal for this recipe because the sauce is white and won't show the specks, but freshly ground black pepper is also fine.

Tahini Sauce

vegan
gluten-free

Tahini is as an easy-to-prepare sauce made from sesame seed paste that can be used in pita sandwiches, marinades, and dips. Store it in an airtight container in the refrigerator and it will keep for about two weeks.

- **2 cloves garlic, peeled**
- **½ cup well-stirred tahini**
- **⅓ cup fresh lemon juice**
- **¼ cup water**
- **1 tbsp. Bragg Liquid Aminos**
- **¼ tsp. cayenne pepper**

1. Place the garlic in the bowl of a food processor and process until minced. Add the remaining ingredients and process until combined well. Makes about 2 cups.

Vegan Worcestershire Sauce

vegan
gluten-free

Most store-bought Worcestershire sauce contains anchovies, making it unfit for vegetarians and vegans. But don't despair; you can make your own anchovy-free version quickly and easily.

- 1½ tsp. dry mustard powder
- 1 tsp. onion powder
- ¾ tsp. ground ginger
- ½ tsp. black pepper
- ¼ tsp. garlic powder
- ¼ tsp. cayenne pepper
- ¼ tsp. ground cinnamon
- ⅛ tsp. cloves or ground allspice
- ⅛ tsp. cardamom powder
- 1 cup cider vinegar
- ⅓ cup molasses
- ¼ cup Bragg Liquid Aminos
- ¼ cup water
- 3 tbsp. lemon juice

1. Place the mustard powder, onion powder, ginger, black pepper, garlic powder, cayenne, cinnamon, cloves or allspice, and cardamom powder in a medium-sized pot. Add the cider vinegar, molasses, Bragg's, water, and lemon juice slowly, stirring constantly.

2. Bring the mixture to a boil over high heat. Reduce the heat to low and simmer, covered, for 5 minutes. The sauce will be very strong-smelling. Cool and store in a jar in the fridge for up to 3 months. Makes about 2 cups.

Spicy Thai Peanut Sauce

vegan
gluten-free

This sauce goes on almost everything. If refrigerated and covered, it may be made up to 3 days ahead. If your sauce is too thick after chilling, stir in 1 to 2 tablespoons of hot water to thin it to the desired consistency.

- 2 cloves garlic, peeled
- 1 (thumb-sized) piece of unpeeled fresh ginger, sliced
- 1 cup water
- ½ cup chunky peanut butter
- 1 tbsp. Bragg Liquid Aminos
- 2 tbsp. brown sugar
- ½ tsp. sambal oelek* or other chili paste
- ¼ tsp. dried red pepper flakes

1. Place the garlic and ginger in the bowl of a food processor and process until minced. Add the remaining ingredients and process to combine. Adjust the seasonings to taste. Makes about 2 cups.

* Sambal oelek is a red chili paste available at most Asian markets.

Zippy Black Bean Sauce

vegan
gluten-free

Serve this sauce with rice, tofu, chicken, or even steamed mussels!

- **3 cloves garlic, minced**
- **I tbsp. grated fresh ginger**
- **I cup black beans, cooked, rinsed, and mashed**
- **2 tbsp. rice vinegar**
- **½ tsp. chili paste**
- **2 tbsp. Bragg Liquid Aminos**
- **2 tbsp. cornstarch**
- **I cup water, divided**
- **I cup orange juice**
- **I tbsp. sesame oil**
- **2 green onions, chopped**

1. Combine the garlic, ginger, and mashed black beans in a small saucepan over medium-high heat. Add the rice vinegar, chili paste, and Bragg's, stirring after each addition.

2. In a small bowl, make a slurry by mixing the cornstarch with ½ cup of the water and stirring until smooth. Pour the slurry into the saucepan and stir to combine. Slowly add the remaining ½ cup of water and the orange juice, stirring constantly. Bring the mixture to a boil and continue to stir for 3 to 5 minutes, or until the liquid thickens.

3. Remove from heat and stir in the sesame oil and green onions. Add more chili paste if you'd like it spicier. Allow to cool and then store in the refrigerator for up to a week. Makes about 3 cups.

Aji Verde

gluten-free

This is a delicious Peruvian green chili salsa sauce. It is lovely as a bread dip or served alongside the Peruvian Roasted Chicken from page 162.

- **2 jalapeño peppers, halved and seeded (wear gloves)**
- **2 cloves garlic, peeled**
- **I bunch cilantro, washed well**
- **½ tsp. sea salt**
- **¼ cup olive oil**
- **2 tbsp. mayonnaise**
- **¼ cup water, if needed**

1. With the food processor running, toss in the peppers and garlic and process until well minced. Add the cilantro leaves and sea salt and blend until combined. Slowly add the olive oil and process until combined. Finally, add the mayonnaise and process until uniform. If the sauce is too thick, slowly add the water until a good dipping consistency is reached. Makes about I cup.

A-1 Aioli Sauce

vegetarian
gluten-free

This fragrant and pungent garlic mayonnaise is excellent with fish. Serve it with grilled salmon, deep fried cod, or baked bass. For some extra flavour, try adding some fresh basil, fennel tops, dill, lemon zest, or my favourite…saffron!

- **2 cloves garlic, peeled**
- **2 room-temperature pasteurized egg yolks***
- **½ tsp. sea salt**
- **½ tsp. freshly ground pepper**
- **1 tbsp. fresh lemon juice**
- **1 tsp. Dijon mustard**
- **1 cup extra virgin olive oil**

1. Place the garlic in the bowl of a food processor and process until minced. Add the egg yolks, sea salt, pepper, lemon juice, and Dijon mustard and process until combined. With the food processor still running, add the olive oil drop by drop. When the sauce begins to thicken, add the remaining oil in a thin stream. Adjust the seasonings and add any flavouring you like, or see the suggestions above. Keeps for 2 or 3 days in the refrigerator. Makes about 1½ cups.

*Unpasteurized raw eggs may contain salmonella. I don't suggest using them in this recipe, since the sauce isn't cooked. You can buy pasteurized eggs at the supermarket or you can pasteurize your own eggs by placing them in a saucepan filled with water over high heat and bringing the water up to 140°F. Keep the water temperature at 140°F (and no more than 142°F) for 3 minutes, reducing the heat on the burner to control the water temperature if necessary. Remove the eggs from the hot water and rinse them thoroughly with cold water. Store them in the refrigerator until needed or use right away.

Garlic Almond Dressing

vegan
gluten-free

This is a nice, simple vegan dressing to go on any type of salad.

- **2 cloves garlic, peeled**
- **12 blanched almonds**
- **½ tsp. sea salt**
- **¼ tsp. cayenne pepper**
- **2 tbsp. white wine vinegar**
- **¼ cup olive oil**

1. Place the garlic in the bowl of a food processor and process until minced. Add the almonds and continue to process until combined. Add the remaining ingredients and blend until smooth. Makes about 1 cup.

Marvellous Mushroom Gravy

vegan
gluten-free

This is a wonderful and easy-to-prepare vegan gravy to serve with potatoes, pasta, or even rice.

- **1 tbsp. sunflower oil**
- **½ cup minced onion**
- **½ cup sliced mushrooms (any variety)**
- **2 cloves garlic, minced**
- **½ tsp. dried rosemary**
- **½ tsp. dried thyme**
- **1½ cups vegetable stock**
- **1 tsp. Bragg Liquid Aminos**
- **2 tbsp. cornstarch**
- **¼ cup water**
- **freshly ground pepper to taste**

1. Place the oil, onions, mushrooms, garlic, and seasonings in a medium saucepan and sauté over medium heat for 4 to 5 minutes, or until the vegetables are soft and the liquid from the mushrooms has evaporated. Add the stock and Bragg's and bring to a boil.

2. In a small bowl, mix the cornstarch and water together to make a slurry. Stir the slurry into the saucepan. Bring the mixture to a boil and then let simmer, uncovered, for 1 minute, stirring occasionally. If the mixture is too thick, slowly add extra water until it reaches the consistency of gravy. Season to taste with freshly ground pepper. Makes about 2 cups.

Herb Marinade

vegan
gluten-free

This is a perfect marinade for meats or vegetables. The longer you marinate them, the better they will be!

- **2 cloves garlic, minced**
- **½ tsp. sea salt**
- **½ tsp. freshly ground pepper**
- **½ tsp. dried basil**
- **½ tsp. dried oregano**
- **½ tsp. dried marjoram**
- **½ tsp. dried rosemary**
- **¼ cup apple cider vinegar**
- **1 tsp. Dijon mustard**
- **¾ cup olive oil**

1. Place all ingredients in a small bowl and mix well to combine. Keep refrigerated until ready to use. Makes about 1 cup.

Orange Tahini Dressing

vegan
gluten-free

Try this dressing on a salad or on fish.

- **2 tsp. tahini**
- **½ tsp. dry mustard powder**
- **I tsp. honey**
- **I orange, zest and juice**
- **I tbsp. balsamic vinegar**
- **½ cup water**
- **¼ tsp. ground cumin**
- **pinch cayenne pepper**

I. Place all of the ingredients in the bowl of a food processor and process until combined well. Keep refrigerated. Makes about I cup.

Maple Salad Dressing

vegan
gluten-free

My friend Val gave me the recipe for this salad dressing many moons ago and I used it well over my catering career. This goes great on any salad, and it can also be used as a marinade.

- **2 tbsp. maple syrup**
- **I tbsp. Dijon mustard**
- **4 tbsp. red wine vinegar**
- **½ cup olive oil**
- **I tbsp. chopped fresh herbs (your choice or what is in season)**
- **I clove garlic, minced**
- **I tsp. Bragg Liquid Aminos**
- **¼ tsp. freshly ground pepper**

I. Place all of the ingredients in a small bowl and combine well. Let stand for I hour before serving. Makes about I cup.

Sweet Onion and Balsamic Relish

vegan
gluten-free

This relish goes wonderfully with our Champion Veggie Burgers (page 122).

- **2 tbsp. olive oil**
- **4 large Vidalia onions, sliced**
- **3 cloves garlic, minced**
- **1 tbsp. fresh or dried rosemary**
- **1 tbsp. balsamic vinegar**
- **1 tbsp. brown sugar**
- **1 tsp. Bragg Liquid Aminos**
- **sea salt to taste**
- **freshly ground pepper to taste**

1. Heat the olive oil in a large skillet over medium heat. Add the onions and sauté for 10 minutes, stirring often. Stir in the garlic and rosemary and sauté for another 3 minutes.

2. Add the balsamic vinegar, brown sugar, and Bragg's and sauté for another 3 minutes, or until it is thick, caramelized, and fragrant. Season to taste with sea salt and freshly ground pepper. Makes about 3 cups. May be stored in the refrigerator for up to 1 week.

Raita

vegetarian
gluten-free

This cucumber and yogurt sauce has a cooling taste that takes away the heat from spicy, hot dishes. It goes well with our Garam Masala and Cashew Chicken (page 148) or Mad for Beef Madras (page 178).

- **½ cucumber, peeled and grated**
- **1 cup natural yogurt**
- **1 tsp. honey**
- **½ lime, juice only**
- **pinch sea salt**
- **pinch chili powder**

1. Place all the ingredients in a medium-sized mixing bowl and stir well to combine. Cover the bowl and refrigerate until ready to serve. Makes about 1½ cups.

Wild Sauce

vegan
gluten-free

This is the sauce that I served at the farmers' market with our Oodles of Noodles (page 94). This recipe was requested many times. It can be also used as a condiment for any meal you want to add some excitement to.

- 1 tbsp. minced garlic
- 1 tbsp. minced fresh unpeeled ginger
- 1 tsp. Patak's hot curry paste
- 1 tbsp. brown sugar
- 1 tbsp. Bragg Liquid Aminos
- ¼ cup lime juice
- ½ cup water

1. Place all the ingredients in a blender or food processor and blend well. Keep refrigerated and shake well before using. Makes about 1 cup.

Mild Sauce

vegan
gluten-free

We also served this sauce with our Oodles of Noodles (page 94) at the farmers' market. It is a little tamer than the wild sauce.

- 1 tbsp. minced fresh garlic
- 1 tbsp. minced fresh unpeeled ginger
- 2 tbsp. brown sugar
- 1 tbsp. cornstarch
- 1 tbsp. Bragg Liquid Aminos
- 1 cup water
- 1 tbsp. sesame oil

1. Combine the garlic, ginger, brown sugar, and cornstarch in a small sauce pan off of the heat. Slowly add the water, stirring constantly. Place the saucepan over medium-high heat. Bring the mixture to a boil and then simmer for 1 minute. Let the sauce cool, then strain out the garlic and ginger. Stir in the sesame oil and mix until combined. Keep refrigerated and shake or stir before using. Makes about 1 cup.

Pepita (Pumpkin Seed) Pesto

vegan
gluten-free

"Pepita" is the Spanish word for pumpkin seed. It sounds much more romantic than the English equivalent, I think. Pepitas are packed with nutrients. They are an excellent source of protein, iron, zinc, manganese, magnesium, phosphorus, copper, and potassium. You can serve this pesto with any type of pasta, smear it on chicken or tofu as a marinade before roasting, or even use it as a dip.

- **1 cup pumpkin seeds, shelled**
- **3 cloves garlic, peeled**
- **1 cup chopped fresh cilantro or parsley**
- **4 green onions, sliced**
- **2 tbsp. fresh lemon juice**
- **⅓ cup olive oil**
- **¼ tsp. salt**

1. Place the pumpkin seeds in a dry skillet over medium heat. Cook, stirring constantly, until they are brown, toasty, and start to pop. Remove to a bowl and set aside.

2. Place the garlic in the bowl of a food processor and process until minced. Add the toasted pumpkin seeds, the cilantro or parsley, the green onions, and the lemon juice and pulse until the mixture is crumbly.

3. With the machine still running, slowly add the olive oil in a thin stream. Blend until the mixture resembles a paste. If the mixture is too thick, blend in some water to thin it out. Add the sea salt and blend to combine. Makes about 2 cups.

Virtuous Vegan Entrées

If you have some vegans in your house or coming for dinner and don't know what to cook for them, don't despair. The following recipes, some made with tofu and some without, are easy to prepare and very tasty. The Vegan Harvest Stew with Herb Dumplings *(page 96)* is savoury and flavourful, while the Spicy Thai Noodles with Tofu and Peanut Sauce *(page 83)* has kick and excitement.

Indonesian Nasi Goreng with Tofu

vegan
gluten-free

Because of the close relationship between Holland and Indonesia from 1602 until 1949, there are many Indonesian influences in Holland. This extended to the food, so since both of my parents are from Holland I was brought up on some great Indonesian fusion. Nasi Goreng, a kind of fried rice, is one of my favourite Indonesian dishes. You can add any vegetables, eggs, or meat you like to it. Here is our tofu version.

- **2 tbsp. Bragg Liquid Aminos**
- **½ cup water**
- **5 cloves garlic, minced, divided**
- **1 (420 g) package firm tofu, pressed* and sliced into finger-sized pieces**
- **1 tbsp. vegetable oil**
- **1 onion, sliced**
- **1 unpeeled carrot, scrubbed and coarsely grated**
- **1 cup mixed colour bell peppers, sliced**
- **1½ tsp. sambal oelek** or Asian chili paste**
- **2 tbsp. ketjap manis*****
- **3 cups cooked brown or white rice**
- **1 cup finely chopped English cucumber**
- **3 green onions, thinly sliced**
- **1 tbsp. lime juice**
- **¼ cup peanuts, roasted and chopped**

1. In a large bowl, combine the Bragg's, water, and 2 cloves of the minced garlic. Add the tofu and toss it in the marinade. Allow the tofu to marinate in the refrigerator from 2 hours to overnight.

2. Cook the marinated tofu by either baking it in a 400°F oven for 15 to 20 minutes or sautéing it in oil over medium-high heat until browned and firm. Set aside.

3. Heat the oil in a large skillet set over medium heat. Add the onion, carrot, bell peppers, and the remaining 3 cloves of garlic and stir-fry until the vegetables are cooked but still have some bite, about 5 minutes. Add the sambal oelek and ketjap manis and stir to combine. Stir in the cooked rice and tofu. Stir-fry until all ingredients are heated through.

4. Garnish with the cucumber, green onions, lime juice, and peanuts. Serves 4.

*For detailed instructions on pressing tofu, see page 10.

**Sambal oelek is a red chili paste available at most Asian markets.

***Ketjap manis is an Indonesian soy sauce that is often sold in grocery stores that cater to an Asian or Dutch clientele. A good substitute for ketjap manis in this recipe is to combine 2 tbsp. Bragg Liquid Aminos with ½ tsp. molasses.

Spicy Fried Tofu

vegan
gluten-free

While we were courting, my husband made this dish for me the first time I went to visit him. It was a winner and now so am I.

- **2 tbsp. sunflower oil**
- **1 (420 g) package firm tofu, pressed***
  and cut into ½-inch cubes
- **½ tsp. ground turmeric**
- **1 tsp. dried dill**
- **½ tsp. dried basil**
- **½ tsp. dried thyme**
- **½ tsp. ground cumin**
- **¾ tsp. curry powder**
- **2 cloves garlic, minced**
- **2 tbsp. Bragg Liquid Aminos**
- **¼ cup nutritional yeast**

1. Heat the oil in a large skillet over high heat. Add the tofu and sauté for 5 minutes, turning the pieces with a spatula. Reduce the heat to medium, add the turmeric, and stir until the tofu is yellow all over.

2. One at a time, add the dill, basil, thyme, cumin, and curry powder, stirring well between each addition. Next add the garlic and more oil if needed to keep the ingredients from sticking to the pan.

3. Add the Bragg's, stirring constantly until combined. Stir in the nutritional yeast and sauté until golden brown. Serve hot or cold. Serves 4 to 6.

*For detailed instructions on pressing tofu, see page 10.

Toasted Tofu and Quinoa Casserole

vegan
gluten-free

Quinoa is one of my favourite grains. It is high in protein and makes an interesting alternative to rice. Quinoa needs to be washed well before cooking to remove the bitter-tasting saponins. I rinse it in a sieve under cold water while stirring it around with my hand for about 5 minutes. After rinsing, if you toast it in a hot dry skillet, it will get a nutty flavour.

- **1 cup uncooked quinoa**
- **1 (420 g) package firm tofu, pressed* and cubed**
- **2 tbsp. vegetable oil, divided**
- **1 onion, diced**
- **2 cloves garlic, minced**
- **1 cup diced squash (any variety) or carrots**
- **1 cup orange or apple juice**
- **1 cup vegetable stock**
- **2 tbsp. Bragg Liquid Aminos**
- **½ cup chopped fresh parsley**

1. Preheat the oven to 375°F.

2. Rinse the quinoa and drain it well. Place the quinoa in a large skillet over medium-high heat and cook, stirring constantly, until all the moisture is gone. Reduce the heat to medium and continue to stir the quinoa until it is lightly toasted. Place the toasted quinoa in a lightly greased baking dish.

3. Place the tofu and 1 tablespoon of the oil in the same large skillet and sauté over medium-high heat until the tofu has browned (about 3 to 4 minutes on each side). Add the tofu to the baking dish and stir to combine with the quinoa.

4. Pour the remaining tablespoon of oil into the skillet. Add the onion and garlic and sauté for 2 to 3 minutes, or until softened. Add the squash or carrots and sauté for 2 to 3 minutes to bring out the sweetness of the squash or carrots. Add the onion mixture, the orange or apple juice, the stock, and the Bragg's to the quinoa and tofu mixture and stir to combine. Cover and bake for 30 minutes.

5. Remove the cover and bake for another 10 minutes, or until the liquid is absorbed and the squash or carrots are tender. Stir in the parsley and fluff with a fork before serving. Serves 4 to 6.

*For detailed instructions on pressing tofu, see page 10.

Spicy Thai Noodles with Tofu and Peanut Sauce

vegan
gluten-free

This was my signature dish when I first started my business. I prepared it at least twice a week. It was quite a challenge for me to adjust the recipe to make it for just the two of us. We would often have leftovers for four days when I tried making it at home!

- **4 tbsp. Bragg Liquid Aminos, divided**
- **½ cup water, divided**
- **5 cloves garlic, minced and divided**
- **3 tbsp. grated fresh unpeeled ginger, divided**
- **1 (420 g) package firm tofu, pressed* and sliced into finger-sized pieces**
- **1 cup crunchy peanut butter**
- **1½ tbsp. brown sugar**
- **1 tsp. cayenne pepper**
- **1 (454 g) package rice vermicelli noodles**
- **2 tbsp. sunflower oil**
- **1 large onion, sliced**
- **4 carrots, peeled and sliced thin diagonally**
- **4 stalks celery, sliced diagonally**
- **1½ cup snow peas or broccoli florets**

1. Combine 2 tablespoons of the Bragg's, ¼ cup of the water, 2 of the cloves of minced garlic, and 1 tablespoon of the grated ginger in a medium-sized bowl. Add the tofu and toss to cover. Set aside in the refrigerator to marinate for at least two hours, stirring occasionally.

2. Preheat the oven to 400°F.

3. Place the peanut butter, brown sugar, cayenne pepper, the remaining ¼ cup of water, and the remaining 2 tablespoons of Bragg's in the bowl of a food processor and blend until combined. Add more water if the mixture is too thick to pour. Set aside.

4. Cook the vermicelli noodles according to the directions on the package. Drain and rinse with cold water. Set aside.

5. Place the marinated tofu on a baking sheet and bake in the preheated oven for 15 to 20 minutes, or until firm. Set aside.

6. Heat the oil in a large skillet or wok over medium-high heat. Add the onion and stir-fry for 3 to 4 minutes, or until they just begin to caramelize. Stirring continually, add the carrots, the remaining ginger and garlic, the celery, and the snow peas or broccoli. Stir-fry for 5 minutes, or until carrots are as soft as you like them. Add the tofu and stir to combine.

7. Reheat the noodles by pouring hot or boiling water over them. Drain and add them to the skillet or wok. Pour the reserved sauce over the top and stir-fry until hot. Adjust the seasonings to taste and add more water if needed. Serves 4 to 6.

*For detailed instructions on pressing tofu, see page 10.

Liz's Tofu Nut Loaf

vegan
gluten-free

In the spring and summer of 2003, we provided catering on a movie set in the northeastern part of PEI. The movie was called The Ballad of Jack and Rose and it starred Daniel Day-Lewis. It was written by Day-Lewis's wife, Rebecca Miller, who is the daughter of the great (now late) Arthur Miller. There were some other notable actors in the movie including Camilla Belle, Catherine Keener, Paul Dano, Jason Lee, Jena Malone, and Beau Bridges. The character that Daniel Day-Lewis played was a vegan, so we needed to make a lot of vegan meals. This dish, which was created by Liz Vaine, who worked in our kitchen, was one of Day-Lewis's favourites.

Serve this with Marvellous Mushroom Gravy (page 74).

- **2 tbsp. ground flaxseed**
- **¼ cup water**
- **1 (420 g) package firm, unpressed tofu**
- **1½ cups cooked brown rice**
- **¾ cup toasted almond pieces**
- **1 tbsp. sunflower oil**
- **1 onion, chopped**
- **1 cup sliced button mushrooms**
- **3 cloves garlic, minced**
- **2 unpeeled carrots, scrubbed and grated**
- **1 tsp. dried rosemary**
- **1 tsp. dried thyme**
- **1 tsp. dried parsley**
- **½ tsp. sea salt**
- **½ tsp. freshly ground pepper**
- **1 tbsp. Bragg Liquid Aminos**

1. Preheat the oven to 350°F.

2. In a small bowl, combine the flaxseed with the water and set aside to soften.

3. Place the tofu in a large bowl and mash it well. Add the cooked rice and toasted almonds and stir to combine. Set aside.

4. Heat the oil in a skillet over medium heat. Add the onion, mushrooms, garlic, carrots, rosemary, thyme, parsley, sea salt, and pepper and sauté for about 5 minutes, or until the vegetables are soft. Add the contents of the skillet to the tofu and rice mixture and stir to combine. Next add the thickened flaxseed mix and the Bragg's and mix well.

5. Pour the batter in a greased loaf pan. Bake for 35 to 45 minutes, or until firm. Let sit for 5 minutes and then turn onto a plate. Slice and serve with mushroom gravy. Serves 4.

Tofu Kohlapuri

vegan
gluten-free

Removing the seeds from the jalapeño peppers tames down the heat a bit—it's your call!

- **1 large onion, roughly chopped**
- **3 to 4 cloves garlic, roughly chopped**
- **1 (1½-inch) piece unpeeled fresh ginger, roughly chopped**
- **1 tbsp. sunflower oil**
- **1 tsp. ground turmeric**
- **2 tsp. ground coriander**
- **1½ tsp. ground cumin**
- **1¼ tsp. chili powder**
- **1 (398 ml) can diced tomatoes**
- **1 (420 g) package firm tofu, pressed* and sliced into 1-inch cubes**
- **1 tsp. Bragg Liquid Aminos**
- **1 cup water**
- **4 to 6 jalapeño peppers, halved and deseeded if desired (wear gloves)**
- **1 tsp. garam masala (page 18)**
- **1 tsp. freshly ground pepper**
- **2 tbsp. chopped fresh cilantro**

1. Place the onion, garlic, and ginger in the bowl of a food processor and blend to a smooth purée.

2. Heat the oil in large pot over medium heat and add the onion purée. Sauté for 2 to 3 minutes, or until soft. Stir in the turmeric, coriander, cumin, and chili powder.

3. Lower the heat to medium and cook for 3 to 4 minutes, stirring frequently. Stir in half the diced tomatoes and cook for 2 to 3 minutes. Next add the tofu and cook at medium heat for 4 to 5 minutes to meld the flavours together.

4. Add the rest of the tomatoes, the Bragg's, and the water. Bring the mixture to a boil, cover, and simmer on low heat for 20 minutes. Stir occasionally to ensure that the sauce doesn't stick to the bottom of the pot. Add the jalapeños and garam masala and cook covered for a further 5 minutes.

5. Stir in the pepper and adjust the seasonings to taste. Garnish with the cilantro and serve with organic brown rice. Serves 4.

*For detailed instructions on pressing tofu, see page 10. If you wish to keep the tofu from falling apart in this dish, you can sear the cubes in a tablespoon of sunflower oil over medium-high heat for 3 to 4 minutes, or until browned.

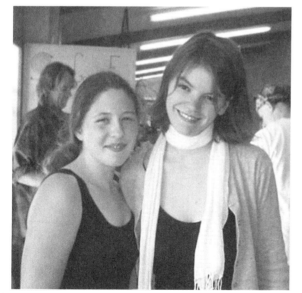

My stepdaughter, Haida (on the right), and her best bud, Chelsea introduced us to this dish. It is now a family favourite

Tahini Tofu

vegan
gluten-free

If you are looking for a tasty calcium boost, try this recipe where sautéed tofu pieces are dipped in tahini sauce and rolled in toasted sesame seeds. Serve this dish with brown rice and broccoli to boost your calcium intake even more.

- **3 tbsp. Bragg Liquid Aminos, divided**
- **½ cup water, divided**
- **1 (420 g) package firm tofu, pressed* and cut into finger-sized slices**
- **2 garlic cloves, peeled**
- **½ cup well-stirred tahini**
- **⅓ cup fresh lemon juice**
- **¼ tsp. cayenne pepper**
- **2 cups sesame seeds**
- **1 to 2 tbsp. sunflower oil**

1. Mix 2 tablespoons of the Bragg's and ¼ cup of the water together in a medium-sized mixing bowl. Add the tofu, coat it in the liquid, and marinate it in the refrigerator for an hour or more.

2. Preheat the oven to 300°F. Put the sesame seeds in a dry skillet and toast over medium-high heat for 4 to 5 minutes, or until golden. Place the seeds in a bowl to cool and set aside.

3. Place the garlic in the bowl of a food processor and process until minced. Add the tahini, lemon juice, cayenne pepper, the remaining ¼ cup of water, and the remaining tablespoon of Bragg's and blend until combined.

4. Remove the tofu from the marinade and set aside. Add the tahini sauce to the remaining marinade and mix well.

5. Warm 1 tablespoon of the oil in the skillet over medium-high heat. Add a few of the tofu pieces and sauté until browned, using more oil if needed. Dip the cooked tofu pieces into the tahini sauce and then roll them in the sesame seeds to coat. Place them on a lightly greased baking sheet and keep them warm in the oven while repeating the cooking and rolling steps with the remaining tofu.

6. Serve with rice or noodles and toss with the remaining tahini sauce. Serves 4.

*For detailed instructions on pressing tofu, see page 10.

Sri Lankan Brinjal Curry

vegan
gluten-free

The Sri Lankans call eggplant "brinjal." You will love the combinations of seasonings used in this curry. If you don't have all the ingredients, go with what you do have. Serve with rice.

- 1 tsp. loosely packed saffron threads
- 2 tbsp. brown mustard seeds
- 1 tbsp. coriander seeds
- 1 tbsp. cumin seeds
- 2 to 3 tbsp. sunflower oil
- 2 medium eggplants, cut into 2-inch cubes and salted*
- 1 large onion, diced
- 4 cloves garlic, minced
- 1 tbsp. grated unpeeled fresh ginger
- 1 tbsp. tamarind paste
- 1 stick lemongrass, chopped finely
- 1 tbsp. curry paste
- 1 medium red chili pepper, seeded and chopped (use gloves)
- 1 tsp. ground cinnamon
- 1 (170 g) can coconut milk
- 1 (796 ml) can diced tomatoes
- 1 tsp. sugar

1. Place the mustard, coriander, and cumin seeds in a dry skillet and toast over medium-high heat for 3 to 5 minutes, or until the seeds are popping and aromatic. Place the toasted seeds in a spice grinder and grind coarsely. Set aside.

2. Rinse the salted eggplant well and pat dry. Heat 1½ tablespoons of the oil in a large skillet over medium-high heat. Add the eggplant and cook, stirring frequently, until it begins to soften, about 4 to 5 minutes. Add the onion, garlic, and ginger to the pan and sauté for another 2 to 3 minutes, or until the onion is soft.

3. Add the toasted spices and the remainder of the ingredients except the sugar and simmer, uncovered, over low heat, stirring frequently, for 15 to 20 minutes, or until the eggplant is very soft.

4. When the curry has finished simmering, stir in the sugar, adjust the seasonings to your taste, and remove it from the heat. Serves 4 to 6.

*For detailed instructions on salting eggplants, see page 17.

Pad Thai with Tofu

vegan
gluten-free

I adjusted this popular dish to make it vegan, gluten-free, and low-fat, but you will still enjoy the harmony of tofu, veggies, fresh lime juice, chili spices, and roasted peanuts.

- **2 limes, zest and juice**
- **1 tbsp. brown sugar**
- **3 cloves garlic, minced**
- **2 tbsp. grated fresh unpeeled ginger**
- **1 tsp. chili flakes**
- **2 tbsp. toasted sesame oil**
- **3 tbsp. Bragg Liquid Aminos**
- **3 tbsp. water**
- **1 (420 g) package firm tofu, pressed* and cut into finger-sized pieces**
- **1 (8 oz.) package Thai rice stick noodles (the flat kind)**
- **2 tbsp. sunflower oil, divided**
- **1 red onion, sliced**
- **1 red bell pepper, sliced into thin strips**
- **1 large unpeeled carrot, scrubbed and grated**
- **3 cups bean sprouts, rinsed and drained**
- **4 green onions, sliced**
- **1 bunch cilantro, washed and chopped**
- **½ cup chopped roasted peanuts**

1. Whisk together the lime zest and juice, brown sugar, garlic, ginger, chili flakes, sesame oil, Bragg's, and water in a small bowl. Place the tofu pieces in a container with a lid. Add about one-third of the sauce to the tofu, seal the container tightly, shake to coat, and set in the refrigerator to marinate. Set the remaining sauce aside.

2. Cook the rice noodles according to the directions on the package. Drain, rinse well with cold water, and set aside.

3. Heat 1 tablespoon of the oil in a large wok over medium-high heat. Remove the tofu from the marinade, reserving the liquid. Add the tofu to the wok in batches, stir-frying until it is fully browned (add extra oil if needed). Remove the tofu from the wok and set aside.

4. Place the remaining tablespoon of oil to the wok and allow it to heat up. Add the onion and sauté for 2 to 3 minutes. Add the red pepper and carrot and stir-fry for another 2 minutes, or until the vegetables are more tender but still crisp. Mix in the reserved tofu and rice noodles, the bean sprouts, and the green onions. Add all the reserved sauce as well as the cilantro and chopped peanuts and toss while stir-frying to reheat. Adjust the seasonings to taste. Serves 4 to 6.

*For detailed instructions on pressing tofu, see page 10.

Southwest Tofu Scramble

vegan
gluten-free

This scramble makes a very nice breakfast. We served it with our homemade salsa (page 68) and our Cornmeal Muffins (page 182) and sold out of it every week at the Charlottetown Farmers' Market. You can also wrap it in a flour tortilla for an easy breakfast burrito.

- **1 tbsp. sunflower oil**
- **1 green bell pepper, diced**
- **1 red bell pepper, diced**
- **1 onion, chopped**
- **8 to 10 button mushrooms, sliced**
- **1 (420 g) package firm tofu, unpressed and mashed**
- **1 tsp. ground turmeric**
- **1 tsp. dried oregano**
- **1 tsp. chili powder**
- **1 tsp. ground cumin**
- **1 tbsp. Bragg Liquid Aminos**
- **2 tbsp. nutritional yeast**

1. Heat the oil in a large skillet over medium-high heat. Add the green and red peppers and the onion and stir-fry for 2 to 3 minutes, or until the vegetables soften. Add the mushrooms and sauté for another 1 to 2 minutes, or until they are soft.

2. Stir in the mashed tofu, turmeric, oregano, chili powder, cumin, Bragg's, and nutritional yeast and stir-fry for 4 to 5 minutes, or until all of the ingredients are well combined. Serve immediately. Serves 4 to 6.

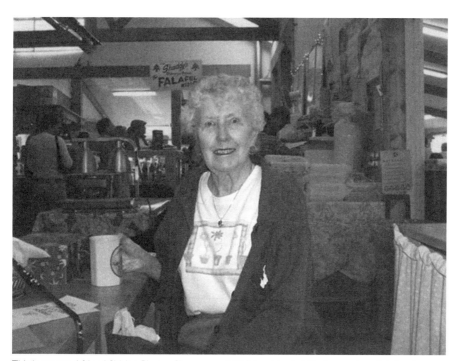

This is my good friend Shirlee Pineau. She was my faithful assistant at the farmers' market for six years.

Sir Paul McCartney's Vegan Enchiladas

vegan

Sir Paul was never physically in our kitchen, but we listened to his music often. This is actually Sir Paul's recipe, and it was a very popular item in the Eat Well kitchen—I could have prepared this every week and always had happy customers!

- **2 large onions, diced, divided**
- **3 cloves garlic, minced, divided**
- **1½ tsp. chili powder, divided**
- **¾ tsp. ground cumin, divided**
- **1 cup tomato sauce**
- **1 cup water**
- **½ tsp. dried oregano**
- **2 tbsp. cornstarch, dissolved in 4 tbsp. water**
- **1 (420 g) package firm tofu, unpressed and mashed**
- **¼ tsp. freshly ground pepper**
- **1½ cups homemade salsa (page 68)**
- **12 large flour tortillas**
- **3 cups steamed spinach, squeezed dry**

1. Preheat the oven to 350°F.

2. Place 1 of the onions, 2 cloves of the garlic, 1 teaspoon of the chili powder, ½ teaspoon of the cumin, the tomato sauce, the water, and the oregano in a small saucepan and cook, covered, over low heat, for 20 minutes.

3. While the sauce is cooking, prepare the filling. In a large bowl, mix the remaining onion, ½ teaspoon chili powder, ¼ teaspoon cumin, and clove of garlic with the tofu, pepper, and salsa. Set aside.

4. Lay out the tortillas and place ¼ cup of the spinach into the middle of each tortilla. Add a scoop of the filling into the middle of each tortilla, dividing it evenly amongst the 12. Fold the tortillas in half, and then fold in the ends. While holding the ends, roll or flip the tortilla over. Place the rolled enchiladas in a baking dish. Set aside.

5. Once the sauce has finished cooking, add the cornstarch mixture into the sauce and stir until combined. Cook until the sauce is thick like salsa.

6. Cover the tortillas with the sauce and bake for 20 to 25 minutes. Serve with Vegan Sour Cream (page 67). Serves 6.

Spice-Crusted Tofu

vegan
gluten-free

This is a quick, easy, and very yummy way to prepare tofu. Serve it with Cumin Rice Pilaf (page 59).

- **3 tbsp. pine nuts**
- **1 tbsp. paprika**
- **1 tsp. ground cumin**
- **1 tsp. ground coriander**
- **½ tsp. sea salt, or to taste**
- **freshly ground pepper to taste**
- **1 (420 g) package extra-firm tofu, pressed* and cut crosswise into 8 slices, ½-inch thick**
- **1 tbsp. sunflower oil**
- **3 tbsp. boiling water**
- **2 tbsp. lemon juice**
- **4 tsp. brown rice syrup**
- **1 tbsp. extra virgin olive oil**

1. Place the pine nuts in a small, dry skillet over medium heat and toast, stirring constantly, for 3 to 5 minutes, or until lightly browned. Set aside to cool.

2. Mix the paprika, cumin, coriander, salt, and pepper in a small bowl. Dredge the tofu pieces liberally with the spice mixture, making sure all sides are coated.

3. Heat the cooking oil in a large skillet over medium-high heat and swirl it around to coat the bottom of the pan evenly. Add the tofu pieces and cook on one side for 4 to 5 minutes, or until they are brown and crusty. Flip the tofu pieces over and cook for another 3 minutes.

4. Stir together the boiling water, lemon juice, brown rice syrup, and extra virgin olive oil in a separate small bowl. Add the brown rice syrup mixture to the pan (it will bubble up and evaporate very quickly) and shake to coat the tofu.

5. Sprinkle the tofu with the toasted pine nuts and serve immediately. Serves 4.

*For detailed instructions on pressing tofu, see page 10.

Holiday Heaven Tofu

vegan
gluten-free

We sold many servings of this tofu during the holidays to families who wanted to offer their vegetarian or vegan members a delicious meal. Serve it with our Savoury Wild Rice, Cranberry, and Almond Pilaf (page 64).

- **1 cup vegetable stock**
- **2 cloves garlic, minced**
- **1 tsp. dried parsley**
- **1 tsp. dried sage**
- **½ tsp. dried rosemary**
- **½ tsp. dried thyme**
- **½ tsp. freshly ground pepper**
- **1 tsp. Bragg Liquid Aminos**
- **1 (420 g) package extra-firm tofu, pressed* and cut into ¼-inch slices**

1. Combine the stock, garlic, parsley, sage, rosemary, thyme, pepper, and Bragg's in a medium-sized mixing bowl. Toss the tofu pieces in the marinade and marinate in the refrigerator from 2 hours to overnight.

2. Preheat the oven to 400°F.

3. Remove the tofu pieces from the marinade and place them on a lightly greased baking sheet. Reserve the remaining marinade liquid.

4. Bake the tofu in the preheated oven for 15 to 20 minutes, occasionally basting them with the reserved marinade. Serves 4.

*For detailed instructions on pressing tofu, see page 10.

Tips for Cooking with Zen

- Embrace the food you are preparing and treat it with respect.
- Buy local.
- Have good music playing while cooking.
- Be silent and present while chopping vegetables.
- Think of who you are preparing this food for and add extra love.
- Be flexible and adventurous. Make it your own.

"Rock Your World" Roasted Ratatouille

vegan
gluten-free

The phrase "too much" doesn't apply to ratatouille if you are fond of this wonderful French dish. Once you've tried it roasted like this, you'll never go back to the traditional cooking method. Not only do the vegetables retain their shape and identity, but they also take on a lovely toasted flavour.

This dish can be served in any number of ways, both hot and cold. Try it as topping for pasta or a filling in an omelette. Or just eat it by itself with a loaf of bread for a Provençal-inspired vegetarian meal.

- 5 to 6 plum tomatoes
- 1 large unpeeled zucchini, sliced in rounds
- 1 large or 2 medium unpeeled eggplants, sliced in rounds and salted*
- 1 red bell pepper, cut into 1-inch squares
- 1 yellow pepper, cut into 1-inch squares
- 2 medium onions, chopped into 1-inch squares
- 5 cloves garlic, finely chopped
- 1 cup thinly sliced fresh basil leaves
- 3 tbsp. olive oil
- 2 tsp. Bragg Liquid Aminos
- 1 tsp. freshly ground pepper
- 1 tsp. dried thyme
- 1 tsp. dried oregano
- ½ tsp. dried rosemary

1. Preheat the oven to 450°F.

2. Place the tomatoes in a large metal bowl or pot. Pour enough boiling water over them to cover them entirely. Leave them for 1 minute, then drain, slip the skins off, and quarter them.

3. Place the tomatoes, zucchini, eggplant, red and yellow peppers, onions, and garlic in a large bowl and toss to combine. Add the basil, olive oil, Bragg's, pepper, thyme, oregano, and rosemary and toss to coat.

4. Arrange the vegetables on a large shallow baking sheet. (Make sure the vegetables aren't crowded—use two sheets if you need them.) Roast the vegetables on the middle shelf of the oven, stirring occasionally, for 30 to 40 minutes (rotating the pans after 20 minutes if you are using two pans), or until the vegetables are tender and tinged brown at the edges. Serves 4 to 6.

*For detailed instructions on salting eggplants, see page 17.

Oodles of Noodles

vegan
gluten-free

Oodles of Noodles were a very popular choice at the farmers' market. Not only was this dish a good, healthy choice, but it was also aesthetically pleasing. We would offer it with nuts and seeds for extra protein and also with the choice of Wild Sauce (page 77) or Mild Sauce (page 77). You can replace the nuts and seeds recommended in this recipe with any nuts and/or seeds of your choice.

- **2 tbsp. white sesame seeds**
- **2 tbsp. black sesame seeds**
- **2 tbsp. sunflower seeds**
- **2 tbsp. pumpkin seeds**
- **2 tbsp. slivered almonds**
- **2 tbsp. cashew pieces**
- **1 (454 g) package rice vermicelli noodles, broken up**
- **2 tbsp. sunflower oil**
- **1 onion, sliced**
- **2 unpeeled carrots, scrubbed and sliced thin on the bias**
- **1 red bell pepper, sliced thin**
- **1 green bell pepper, sliced thin**
- **2 stalks celery, sliced thin on the bias**
- **2 cups snow peas or sugar snap peas,**
- **trimmed and strings removed***
- **2 cups mung bean sprouts, well rinsed**

1. Place the white and black sesame seeds in a skillet over medium-high heat. Stir or shake the pan constantly for 3 to 4 minutes, or until the seeds darken and become fragrant. Pour the toasted seeds into a bowl to cool and set aside.

2. Add the sunflower seeds, pumpkin seeds, slivered almonds, and cashew pieces to the same skillet with the heat still at medium-high. Toast them, stirring constantly, for 4 to 5 minutes, or until they are lightly browned. Pour them into a separate bowl to cool and set aside.

3. Bring a large pot of water to a boil over medium-high heat. Add the rice vermicelli noodles and cook, uncovered, for 3 minutes. Drain, rinse the noodles well with cold water, and set aside.

4. Heat the oil in a large skillet or wok over medium-high heat. Add the onion, carrots, red and green pepper, celery, and peas and stir-fry for 5 to 6 minutes, or until the vegetables are al dente and still have their bright colors. (Pick up a piece of snow pea or pepper and test the texture.) Add the bean sprouts and stir-fry until hot. Be careful not to overcook the vegetables. Remove the vegetables from heat and set aside.

5. Reheat the rice noodles by soaking them in hot or boiling water for 2 to 3 minutes. Drain.

6. Serve the Oodles of Noodles by placing 1 cup of noodles in a bowl, topping the noodles with ½ to ¾ cup of the cooked vegetable mixture, and then adding 2 tablespoons (depending on your taste) of Wild Sauce (page 77) or Mild Sauce (page 77). Sprinkle 1 tablespoon of the toasted nut and seed mixture and ¾ tablespoon of the sesame seeds on top. Serves 6.

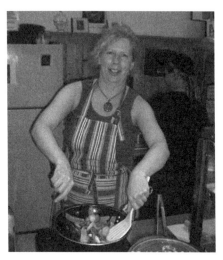

Stirring up the Oodles of Noodles at the farmers' market.

*Snow and sugar snap peas are delicious, but they have little strings running up both sides of each pea, which aren't pleasant to eat.. We use a sharp paring knife to trim the top of the pea and remove the string down one side and then trim the bottom and remove the string from the other side.

Peanut Millet with Roasted Curried Vegetables

vegan
gluten-free

Millet is a popular bird food, but it's great for humans too. It is a small, round, yellow grain with a tiny dot on one side that is nutritious and gluten-free. When prepared this way, it makes a tasty vegan meal with lots of protein, veggies, and flavour.

- 2 red onions, cut into thumb-sized pieces
- 3 unpeeled carrots, scrubbed and cut into thumb-sized pieces
- 1 eggplant, cut into thumb-sized pieces and salted*
- 1 red bell pepper, cut into thumb-sized pieces
- 1 green bell pepper, cut into thumb-sized pieces
- 8 to 10 small button mushrooms
- 3 tbsp. olive oil
- 3 tbsp. balsamic vinegar
- 2 tbsp. orange juice
- 2 cloves garlic, minced
- 1 tbsp. grated unpeeled fresh ginger
- 2 tbsp. curry powder
- ½ tsp. ground cinnamon
- 1 tbsp. brown rice syrup
- sea salt to taste
- freshly ground pepper to taste
- 1 cup uncooked millet
- 2 cups water
- 1 cup peanuts, toasted and chopped
- ½ tbsp. Bragg Liquid Aminos

1. Place the onions, carrots, eggplant, red and green peppers, and mushrooms in a large bowl and toss to combine.

2. In a separate small bowl, combine the olive oil, balsamic vinegar, orange juice, garlic, ginger, curry powder, cinnamon, brown rice syrup, salt, and pepper. Pour the marinade over the vegetables and mix well so all the vegetables are coated. Set aside and let sit for 2 to 6 hours or longer.

3. Preheat the oven to 425°F.

4. Spread the vegetables out on one or two baking sheets, making sure not to crowd them. Roast in the preheated oven for 35 to 40 minutes, or until the vegetables are cooked through and browned, stirring every 10 minutes.

5. While the vegetables are roasting, rinse the millet in a sieve, and then place it in a medium-sized saucepan over high heat. Stir constantly until the millet starts popping, but take care to ensure that it doesn't burn. Add the water to the pot, bring to a boil, cover, and let simmer on low heat for 25 minutes, or until all the liquid has been absorbed.

6. Stir in the peanuts and the Bragg's and serve topped with the warm roasted veggies. Serves 4.

*For detailed instructions on salting eggplants, see page 17.

Vegan Harvest Stew with Herb Dumplings

vegan

This stew is a delicious, homey comfort food. You can substitute the vegetables in the recipe for whatever you have in your fridge or whatever is in season—just be sure they are cut in uniform sizes.

- ½ cup whole wheat flour
- ½ cup unbleached white flour
- 2 tsp. baking powder
- 1 tsp. salt, divided
- 1 tsp. apple cider vinegar
- 1 cup soy milk
- 2 tbsp. Earth Balance margarine or other vegan margarine
- 1 tbsp. fresh or dried chives
- 3 tsp. dried thyme, divided
- 2 pears, peeled, cored and cut into pieces
- 2 cups vegetable stock
- 1 tbsp. Dijon mustard
- freshly ground pepper
- 2 tbsp. sunflower oil
- 1 large onion, sliced
- 4 cloves garlic, minced
- 2 small sweet potatoes, peeled and cut into cubes
- 3 carrots, peeled and cut into 1-inch pieces
- 3 parsnips, peeled and cut into 1-inch pieces
- 2 zucchinis, sliced

1. Combine the whole wheat and white flours, baking powder, and ½ teaspoon of the salt in a large bowl.

2. In a separate small bowl, combine the vinegar and the soy milk to curdle. Add the melted margarine and mix to combine. Add the butter and milk mixture to flour mixture and stir until it forms a soft dough. Mix in the chives and 1 teaspoon of the thyme. Set aside.

3. Place the pears in the bowl of a food processor and process until they are puréed. Add the stock, mustard, pepper, the remaining ½ teaspoon of salt, and the remaining 2 teaspoons of thyme and process until combined. Set aside.

4. In a large pot, heat the oil over medium heat. Add the onion and garlic and sauté for 2 to 3 minutes. Next add the sweet potatoes, carrots, parsnips, and zucchinis and sauté for another 2 to 3 minutes, or until the vegetables begin to soften. Pour in the stock mixture and bring to a boil. Adjust the seasonings to taste.

5. Drop the dumpling dough onto the stew by heaping tablespoons. Reduce the heat to medium-low and simmer, uncovered, for 10 minutes. Then cover and cook for another 10 minutes, or until the dumplings are firm. Serves 4.

Vegan Paella Española

vegan
gluten-free

This vegan paella is so moist, full of flavour, and substantial that you will scarcely notice it is meat-free. The tangy artichoke hearts, delicate peas, and juicy tomatoes ensure that this vegetarian paella will satisfy even the most avid carnivores.

- **4 cups vegetable stock**
- **large pinch saffron**
- **2 tbsp. plus 1 tsp. sunflower oil, divided**
- **1 large onion, diced**
- **3 cloves garlic, minced**
- **2½ cups halved button mushrooms**
- **1 yellow pepper, diced**
- **1 green bell pepper, diced**
- **1½ cups uncooked brown rice**
- **1 (796 ml) can diced tomatoes**
- **1 tsp. ground turmeric**
- **1 tsp. smoked paprika or chipotle pepper**
- **1 tsp. fennel seeds**
- **1 tbsp. Bragg Liquid Aminos**
- **freshly ground pepper**
- **1 cup sugar snap peas**
- **1 cup marinated artichoke hearts, sliced**

1. In a large pot, heat the stock to boiling. Remove from the heat and add the saffron. Set aside.

2. Heat 2 tablespoons of the oil in a large skillet or wok over medium-high heat. Add the onion and garlic and stir-fry for 2 to 3 minutes. Next add the mushrooms and yellow and green peppers and stir-fry for 1 to 2 minutes.

3. Turn the heat up to high and add the stock, rice, tomatoes, turmeric, paprika or chipotle, fennel seeds, and Bragg's and bring to a boil. Cover, reduce the heat to low, and simmer, without stirring, for 40 minutes, or until the rice is tender.

4. While the paella is simmering, heat the remaining 1 teaspoon of oil in a small pan over medium-high heat. Add the snow peas and sauté for 2 to 3 minutes, or until slightly tender. Once the paella has finished simmering, add the snow peas and artichokes and cook for 4 to 5 more minutes. Adjust the seasonings to taste. Serves 6.

Egyptian Bean and Vegetable Stew

vegan
gluten-free

This recipe has yummy seasonings and lots of great vegetables. Serve it with rice or pita bread.

- **2 tbsp. olive oil**
- **1 onion, diced**
- **4 cloves garlic, peeled**
- **1 tsp. sea salt**
- **2 to 3 medium unpeeled potatoes, washed and sliced**
- **3 tbsp. lemon juice**
- **1 tsp. ground cinnamon**
- **1 tsp. ground coriander**
- **1 bay leaf**
- **½ tsp. freshly ground pepper**
- **¼ tsp. crushed chili peppers**
- **2 unpeeled carrots, scrubbed and sliced thin**
- **1 small cauliflower, cut into florets**
- **3 large tomatoes, diced**
- **2 tsp. brown rice syrup or brown sugar**
- **2 cups red or white kidney beans, cooked and rinsed**

1. Heat the olive oil in large pot over medium heat. Add the onion, garlic, and salt and sauté for 2 to 3 minutes. Add the potato slices and lemon juice. Cover the pot and cook for 8 to 10 minutes, stirring occasionally. Add a little water if the potatoes stick to the pot.

2. Stir in the cinnamon, coriander, bay leaf, pepper, chili peppers, carrots, cauliflower florets, tomatoes, and brown rice syrup or brown sugar. Cover and simmer over low heat for 30 minutes, stirring occasionally. Add the cooked beans, stir, and simmer for 10 more minutes. Serves 4 to 6.

Asparagus, Dill, and Almond Risotto

vegan
gluten-free

This is a great meal to celebrate the arrival of spring, when the asparagus is in season. The lemon adds some extra freshness and flavour. If you would like to add extra colour, sauté half a diced red bell pepper with the asparagus. For more tips on cooking risotto, see page 19.

- **1 lb. asparagus**
- **3 tbsp. olive oil, divided**
- **4 cloves garlic, minced**
- **¼ cup water**
- **sea salt to taste**
- **freshly ground pepper to taste**
- **½ tsp. freshly ground pepper**
- **4 cups vegetable stock**
- **1 tbsp. Bragg Liquid Aminos**
- **1 red onion, minced**
- **1 cup uncooked arborio rice**
- **½ cup white wine**
- **zest of 1 lemon, minced**
- **2 tbsp. fresh dill, finely chopped**
- **½ cup slivered almonds, toasted**

1. Break off the woody ends from the asparagus and discard. Cut off the asparagus tops and reserve. Chop the remaining stems into pieces.

2. Heat 1 tablespoon of the oil in a sauté pan over medium-high heat. Add the stem pieces and cook for 2 minutes. Stir in 2 cloves of the garlic and the asparagus tips. Pour the water over the asparagus and season with salt and pepper to taste. Cook for 2 to 3 minutes, or until the asparagus is still slightly firm. Set aside.

3. In a large saucepan over medium-high heat, bring the stock and Bragg's to a boil. Reduce the heat to low and simmer until needed.

4. Heat the remaining 2 tablespoons of oil in a large saucepan over medium-high heat. Add the onion and garlic and cook, stirring with a wooden spoon, for 2 to 3 minutes, or until soft.

5. Add the rice and stir until translucent, about 4 minutes. Stir in the wine and reduce until almost dry.

6. Add a ladle of the heated stock and cook, stirring constantly, until the rice absorbs it. Continue adding the stock a ladle at a time and stirring constantly until the rice is tender and creamy, about 20 to 25 minutes. Stop when the rice is al dente, cooked to the bite.

7. Stir in the asparagus, lemon zest, dill, and toasted almonds. Adjust the seasonings to taste. Serves 4.

Curried Squash, Wild Rice, & Apricot Pilaf

vegan
gluten-free

Not only is this meal filled with attractive textures and flavours, it also offers you a powerhouse of nutrition. In other words…it is pretty, tasty, and good for you!

- 1 tsp. sunflower oil
- 1 large onion, diced
- 2 tsp. minced garlic
- 2 tsp. curry powder
- 1 cup uncooked wild rice
- 1 cup uncooked organic brown rice
- 4 cups vegetable stock
- 1 bay leaf
- 1 tsp. Bragg Liquid Aminos
- ½ tsp. sea salt
- ½ tsp. freshly ground pepper
- 1½ cups squash or sweet potatoes, peeled and diced
- ½ cup chopped dried apricots
- ½ cup slivered almonds, toasted
- 2 tbsp. chopped fresh parsley

1. Heat the oil in a large saucepan over medium-high heat. Stir in the onion, garlic, and curry powder. Sauté for 3 to 4 minutes, or until the onions are soft.

2. Rinse the wild and brown rices and add them to the onion mixture. Cook, stirring constantly, for another 2 minutes. Add the stock, bay leaf, Bragg's, sea salt, and pepper and bring to a boil. Simmer, covered, on low heat for 30 minutes without stirring.

3. Add the squash or sweet potatoes and cook for another 10 minutes, or until the squash is tender and the liquid is absorbed. Gently stir in the apricots, almonds, and fresh parsley. Let stand, covered, for 10 minutes before serving. Serves 4 to 6.

Meatless and Manageable

The recipes in this chapter are meatless, but may contain eggs, cheese, or milk. They are also quite easy to prepare. If you love quiche but dislike making crust, you will love our "It's So Easy" Vegetable and Cheese Pie *(page 103)*. The Potato, Sweet Potato, and Gruyère Pie *(page 112)* shows you that working with phyllo is much easier than you thought. We have also included one of my favourite meatless meals: Zesty Baked Eggplant Parmesan *(page 110)*!

Herb Risotto with Pipérade

vegetarian with vegan option
gluten-free

Pipérade is a dish from the Basque region of France. It features tomatoes and green bell peppers cooked in olive oil. Make it first, and keep it warm while you prepare the risotto.

For the vegan option, omit the Parmesan cheese from the risotto.

Pipérade

- **2 tbsp. olive oil**
- **1 large onion, diced**
- **1 cup coarsely chopped bell peppers (preferably a mix of red, yellow, and green)**
- **3 garlic cloves, minced**
- **2 large plum tomatoes, seeded and coarsely chopped**
- **sea salt to taste**
- **freshly ground pepper to taste**

1. Heat the oil in a large skillet over medium-high heat. Add the onion, bell peppers, and garlic and sauté until the vegetables begin to soften, about 5 minutes. Add the tomatoes and sauté for 3 more minutes, or until the tomatoes are falling apart. Season to taste with salt and pepper.

Risotto*

- **3 cups vegetable stock**
- **1½ tbsp. olive oil**
- **1 onion, chopped**
- **2 cloves garlic, minced**
- **2 cups uncooked arborio rice**
- **½ cup dry white wine**
- **sea salt to taste**
- **freshly ground pepper to taste**
- **½ cup grated Parmesan cheese****

1. Place the stock in a saucepan over medium heat and cook until heated through. Keep the stock warm while continuing to prepare the rest of the dish.

2. Heat the olive oil in a large skillet over medium-high heat. Add the onion and garlic and sauté for 2 to 3 minutes, or until the onions have a nice golden appearance.

3. Stir in the rice and make sure it is evenly coated in the olive oil. Gently toast the rice, stirring constantly, for 2 to 3 minutes. Stir in the white wine.

4. Reduce the heat to low. Add 1 ladle of the stock, or enough so that the rice stays wet but is not completely covered by the broth, and stir constantly until the rice has absorbed the liquid. Add another ladle of stock and repeat this step until the grains are tender but still firm to the bite (al dente).

5. When the rice is cooked, season it with salt and pepper to taste and stir in the Parmesan cheese if desired. Serve with the warm pipérade. Serves 4.

*For more tips on cooking risotto, see page 19.

**Optional.

"It's So Easy" Vegetable and Cheese Pie

vegetarian

Impress your friends with this simple yet attractive dish. It is easier to make than quiche and perhaps even tastier. Use your favourite vegetables or whatever is in season.

- **1 tbsp. sunflower oil**
- **1 red onion, sliced**
- **2 cloves garlic, minced**
- **1 red bell pepper, sliced**
- **1 tbsp. fresh dill or 1 tsp. dry dill**
- **½ tsp. sea salt**
- **¼ tsp. freshly ground pepper**
- **2 cups chopped vegetables of your choice (broccoli, cauliflower, mushrooms, cooked spinach, etc.)**
- **½ cup low-fat herbed cream cheese**
- **1 cup whole wheat flour**
- **2 tsp. baking powder**
- **¼ cup butter, chilled and cubed**
- **4 eggs, beaten**
- **1½ cups low-fat or skim milk**
- **1½ cups of your choice of grated cheese, divided**

1. Preheat the oven to 350°F.

2. Heat the oil in a large skillet over medium heat. Add the onion, red pepper, and garlic and sauté for 2 to 3 minutes. Stir in the dill, salt, pepper, and chopped vegetables and sauté for 3 to 4 minutes, or until the vegetables are slightly soft.

3. Pour the vegetable mixture into a lightly greased 10-inch pie pan. Decorate the top with teaspoons of the cream cheese and set aside.

4. In a large bowl, combine the flour with the baking powder. Using a pastry blender or two knives, cut in the butter and combine until the mixture is crumbly. Add the eggs, milk, and ¾ cup of the grated cheese and stir until smooth.

5. Pour the batter over the vegetables in the pie pan. Bring some of the more colourful vegetables to the top for a nice presentation and sprinkle the remaining ¾ cup of cheese over the top.

6. Bake for about 45 minutes, or until golden and your knife comes out clean after being inserted. Let stand for 5 minutes before serving. Serves 4 to 6

"It's So Easy" Vegetable and Cheese Pie

Ken's "Full of Cheese" Veggie Squares

gluten-free

When my son Ken became a vegetarian, he created this recipe. As you can tell, he is a lover of cheese, but judging by the popularity of this meal with the Eat Well customers, there are many more cheese lovers out there. If you have a food processor, you can use it to grate the cheese and slice, mince, or grate the vegetables.

- 2 or 3 sweet potatoes, peeled and sliced
- 2 tbsp. sunflower oil
- 2 medium onions, sliced
- 3 to 4 cloves garlic, minced
- 4 unpeeled carrots, scrubbed and grated
- 3 to 4 zucchinis, grated
- 10 to 12 button mushrooms, sliced
- 1 green bell pepper, sliced
- 1 (10 oz.) package frozen chopped spinach, thawed and well drained
- 1 cup Eat Well Tomato Sauce (page 67) or store-bought tomato sauce
- 1 tsp. sea salt
- 1 tsp. freshly ground pepper
- 1 cup grated mozzarella cheese
- 1 cup grated cheddar cheese
- 1 cup crumbled feta or goat cheese
- ½ cup grated Parmesan cheese

1. Preheat the oven to 350°F.

2. Place the sweet potatoes in a large saucepan and cover them with water. Bring to a boil over high heat and cook for 4 to 5 minutes, or until soft. Drain and set aside.

3. Heat the oil in a large skillet over medium-high heat. Add the onions and stir-fry for 2 to 3 minutes, or until soft. Add the garlic, carrots, zucchinis, mushroom, green pepper, and spinach, stirring between each addition, and sauté for another 4 to 5 minutes, or until the vegetables are tender.

4. Add the tomato sauce, salt, pepper, and the cooked sweet potatoes and stir gently to combine.

5. Pour the mixture onto a lightly greased baking sheet with sides and spread to the edges. Sprinkle the mozzarella over the vegetable mixture in an even layer, then the cheddar, then the feta or goat cheese, and finally the Parmesan, making sure the vegetable mixture is completely covered with cheese.

6. Bake in the preheated oven for 30 to 35 minutes, or until the cheeses are golden brown and melted. Remove from oven and let stand for 5 minutes before slicing. Using a pizza cutter or knife, slice into squares with two vertical cuts and two horizontal cuts. Serves 4 (1 serving is 2 pieces).

Shakshouka

vegetarian
gluten-free

This Tunisian and Israeli dish is a staple traditionally served at breakfast in a cast iron pan with bread to mop up the sauce. This is a terrific way to start your day. "Bete'avon!"(Hebrew for bon appétit).

- **3 tbsp. olive oil**
- **2 onions, chopped**
- **4 cloves garlic, minced**
- **1 green bell pepper, sliced thin**
- **1 red bell pepper, sliced thin**
- **3 cups diced tomatoes**
- **1 tsp. ground cumin**
- **1 tsp. paprika**
- **1 tsp. sea salt**
- **1 tsp. freshly ground pepper**
- **½ tsp. cayenne pepper**
- **6 eggs**

1. Heat the olive oil in a large cast-iron frying pan or skillet over medium heat. Stir in the onions, garlic, and green and red peppers. Sauté until the vegetables have softened and the onions have turned translucent, about 5 minutes.

2. Pour the tomatoes, cumin, paprika, salt, pepper, and cayenne pepper into the skillet and stir to combine. Reduce the heat to low and simmer, uncovered, until the tomato juices have cooked off, about 10 minutes.

3. Make 6 indentations in the tomato mixture for the eggs. Crack the eggs into the indentations. Cover the skillet and let the eggs cook until they're firm but not dry, about 5 minutes.

4. Serve with bread or rice. Serves 4 to 6.

Vegetable Upside-Down Cake

vegetarian

Here is something a little different that will spark conversation at a potluck. I can't remember where this recipe came from, but it was popular with our Eat Well clients. The recipe calls for cooked vegetables. I usually used roasted vegetables, ratatouille, or whatever was in season. This was my friend Amy's favourite.

- **1 ½ cups unbleached white flour**
- **1 ½ cups whole wheat flour**
- **1 cup cornmeal**
- **4 tsp. baking powder**
- **½ cup butter, softened**
- **2 cups milk**
- **2 eggs, beaten**
- **2 tbsp. honey**
- **6 cups cooked vegetables**
- **crumbled feta cheese, chopped nuts, or diced tomatoes for garnish***

1. Preheat the oven to 400°F.

2. Combine the white and whole wheat flours, cornmeal, and baking powder in a large bowl. Cut in the butter until it is the size of peas.

3. In a separate small bowl, mix the milk, eggs, and honey together. Add the milk mixture to the flour mixture and stir until it forms a thick, smooth batter.

4. Arrange the vegetables in an attractive pattern in the bottom of a lightly greased 9" × 13" baking pan. Pour the batter evenly over the vegetables.

5. Bake for 20 to 25 minutes, or until a knife inserted in the centre comes out clean. Invert the cake onto a platter. Garnish with your choice of feta cheese, chopped nuts, or diced tomatoes. Serves 6 to 8.

*Optional

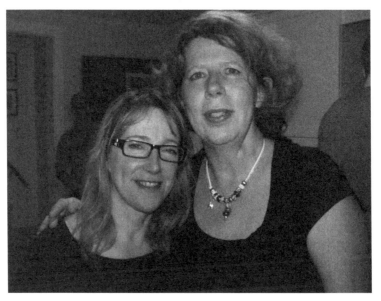

Amy has been a great supporter of my business and also of me since I've been ill. She is awesome!

Moroccan Spinach and Rice Pie

vegetarian
gluten-free

This is a nice vegetarian and gluten-free treat incorporating lovely Moroccan flavours.

- 1 (250 g) container cottage cheese
- 2 cups cooked organic brown rice, cooled
- 1 lemon, zest and juice
- 1 tbsp. sunflower oil
- 1 large onion, sliced
- 3 cloves garlic, minced
- 1 (300 g) package frozen spinach, thawed and drained
- ½ tsp. ground cinnamon
- ½ cup raisins
- 2 cups Eat Well Tomato Sauce (page 67)
- 3 cups shredded mozzarella cheese, divided

1. Preheat the oven to 350°F.

2. Using a hand blender or food processor, blend the cottage cheese until smooth. In a large bowl, combine the blended cottage cheese with the organic brown rice and the zest and juice of the lemon. Press into a 9-inch pie pan to form a crust. Set aside.

3. Heat the oil in large skillet over medium-high heat. Add the onion and the garlic and sauté for 5 minutes, or until browned. Add the spinach, cinnamon, and raisins and stir until well mixed. Next add the tomato sauce and 1 cup of the shredded mozzarella cheese and stir again to combine.

4. Pour the mixture onto the crust in the pie pan and sprinkle the top with the remaining mozzarella cheese. Bake for 30 to 35 minutes, or until golden brown. Serves 4 to 6.

Ginny Callan's Greek Spinach-Potato Strudel

vegetarian

Ginny Callan is a wonderful vegetarian cookbook writer from Vermont. I saw this recipe in one of her cookbooks and I knew it was a winner. We changed it up a bit by adding some sweet potatoes to the mix. The strudel is made of phyllo dough stuffed with potatoes, sweet potatoes, cheese, and seasoning. Don't let the word "phyllo" intimidate you—it is friendly to work with.

- **6 cups diced unpeeled white and sweet potatoes**
- **5 tbsp. butter, divided**
- **1 (10 oz) package frozen spinach, thawed and thoroughly drained**
- **2 tbsp. sunflower oil**
- **3 onions, chopped**
- **5 garlic cloves, minced**
- **2 tsp. dried basil**
- **2 tsp. dried thyme**
- **2 tsp. dried or ¼ cup minced fresh dill, divided**
- **¼ tsp. ground nutmeg**
- **1 tsp. sea salt**
- **½ tsp. freshly ground pepper**
- **¾ cup low-fat sour cream**
- **1½ cups crumbled feta or goat cheese**
- **1 cup grated cheddar cheese**
- **6 green onions, sliced and divided**
- **10 sheets phyllo dough***

1. Place the potatoes in a large pot and cover with water. Bring to a boil over high heat and cook until tender, about 20 to 25 minutes. Drain and remove to a large mixing bowl. Add 1 tablespoon of the butter and mash until smooth. Stir in the spinach and set aside.

2. Heat the oil in a skillet over medium heat. Add the onions, garlic, basil, thyme, and dill (if using dried dill) and sauté until the onions are soft, about 5 minutes. Stir the onion mixture into the potato and spinach mixture. Add the nutmeg, sea salt, pepper, sour cream, feta or goat cheese, cheddar, and all but 1 tablespoon of the fresh dill (if using fresh dill) and green onions and mix well using your hands if needed. Set the filling aside.

3. Preheat the oven to 375°F.

4. Melt the remaining 4 tablespoons of the butter in a small saucepan over medium heat. Spread a single sheet of phyllo dough out on a clean work surface and brush it evenly with butter. Stack four more sheets of phyllo dough on top, brushing each with butter before adding the next layer.

5. Spread half the filling lengthwise over one side of the dough, covering one third of the dough and leaving a 2-inch border on the three outside edges. Fold those edges up over the filling and then roll the filling over the empty dough so it forms a log shape. Gently place the filled dough on an ungreased baking sheet. Repeat the previous steps with the remaining dough sheets and filling.

6. Brush each log with the remaining melted butter. Bake in the preheated oven for 15 to 20 minutes, or until golden. Serves 6.

*You can buy phyllo dough in the freezer section of any large grocery store. Let the phyllo thaw in your fridge overnight before you use it.

Vegetable Strata with Gruyère

vegetarian
gluten-free

Looking for a brunch idea? Try this strata. Most stratas use bread, but we thought we would make it gluten-free by using potatoes instead.

- **4 large unpeeled potatoes, sliced thin**
- **1 tbsp. sunflower oil**
- **1 onion, diced**
- **3 cloves garlic, minced**
- **2 zucchinis, sliced thin**
- **12 plum tomatoes, cut into ½-inch slices**
- **½ tsp. dried oregano**
- **½ tsp. dried basil**
- **1 tsp. sea salt**
- **½ tsp. freshly ground pepper**
- **1 cup grated Gruyère cheese**
- **10 fresh basil leaves, coarsely chopped**

1. Place the sliced potatoes in a large saucepan and cover with water. Bring to a boil over high heat and cook for 10 minutes, or until tender but not crumbling. Drain and set aside.

2. Preheat the oven to 425°F.

3. Heat the oil in a medium-sized skillet over medium-high heat. Add the onions and garlic and stir-fry 4 to 5 minutes, or until lightly browned. Set aside.

4. Place half of the potatoes in a single layer in the bottom of a 9" × 13" baking dish. Place half the zucchini slices in a singer layer on top, and then half the tomato slices on a third layer. Sprinkle with half the dried oregano, dried basil, salt, and pepper. Repeat the layering steps with the remaining potatoes, zucchini, tomatoes, and herbs.

5. Sprinkle the onion and garlic mixture over the layered vegetables. Cover evenly with the grated Gruyère. Place in the preheated oven and bake, uncovered, for 45 to 50 minutes, or until a fork goes through the vegetables easily. Sprinkle the fresh basil over dish before serving. Serves 6 to 8.

Zesty Baked Eggplant Parmesan

vegetarian

I'm a big fan of this warm, belly-filling, Italian comfort-food dish. Our healthy, no-fry, guilt-free version is much more enjoyable than the original fried version.

- **3 cups wheat germ**
- **1 cup Parmesan cheese, divided**
- **2 tsp. dried Italian seasoning**
- **2 large eggs**
- **2 garlic cloves, minced**
- **1 large eggplant, peeled, cut into ¼-inch slices, and salted***
- **4 cups Eat Well Tomato Sauce (page 67)**
- **1 tsp. crushed red pepper flakes**
- **1 cup shredded part-skim mozzarella cheese**

1. Preheat the oven to 400°F.

2. In a shallow dish, combine the wheat germ, ½ cup of the Parmesan cheese, and the Italian seasoning. Set aside.

3. In separate shallow dish, beat the eggs and stir in the minced garlic. Set aside.

4. Rinse the eggplant slices to remove the excess salt from the salting process and pat them dry with paper towels. Dip each eggplant slice into the egg mixture and then immediately dredge in the wheat germ mix until evenly coated. Place the breaded eggplant slices on a lightly greased baking sheet. Bake in the preheated oven for 15 minutes or until golden. Set aside.

5. Reduce the oven temperature to 375°F.

6. In a large bowl, combine the tomato sauce and the red pepper flakes. Spread ½ cup of the tomato sauce evenly over the bottom of a lightly greased 9" × 13" baking dish.

7. Arrange the eggplant slices in layers over the sauce. Spread the remaining tomato sauce over the eggplant. Sprinkle the mozzarella cheese and the remaining Parmesan cheese evenly on top.

8. Bake for 25 minutes, or until the sauce is bubbly and the cheese has melted. Serves 4 to 6.

*For detailed instructions on salting eggplants, see page 17.

Mexican Spinach and Mushroom Frittata

vegetarian
gluten-free

This frittata is one of my good friend Ellie's favourites, and it has super health powers—the spinach used in this recipe is packed with vitamins, minerals, and antioxidants.

- **1 tbsp. sunflower oil**
- **1½ cups sliced mushrooms**
- **½ cup finely chopped green onions**
- **2 cloves garlic, minced**
- **4 eggs or equivalent egg substitute**
- **1 (10 ounce) package frozen chopped spinach, thawed and drained**
- **1 cup low-fat cottage cheese**
- **½ tsp. ground cumin**
- **½ tsp. chili powder**
- **½ tsp. sea salt**
- **½ tsp. freshly ground pepper**
- **1½ cups homemade salsa (page 68)**

1. Preheat the oven to 375°F.

2. Heat the oil in an ovenproof skillet over medium-high heat. Add the mushrooms, green onions, and garlic and sauté for 4 to 5 minutes, or until the mushrooms are soft. Turn off the heat.

3. In a large bowl, whisk together the eggs, spinach, cottage cheese, cumin, sea salt, and pepper. Add the egg mixture to the sautéed vegetables and stir to combine.

4. Bake for 30 minutes, or until browned and set. Let cool for 10 minutes, cut in wedges, and serve with salsa. Serves 4.

Potato, Sweet Potato, and Gruyère Pie

vegetarian

My son Elliot loves this pie. He asked for this for his birthday this year.

Using phyllo dough as a crust means that this pie takes no longer to prepare than a pie with a typical pastry crust, and the results are spectacular! You can find phyllo near the frozen pie shells in the freezer section of any large grocery store. Let the phyllo thaw in your fridge overnight before you use it.

- **2 cloves garlic, finely minced**
- **I cup finely chopped green onions**
- **I tsp. dry rosemary or I tbsp. fresh rosemary**
- **4 medium unpeeled Yukon Gold or Russet potatoes, sliced very thin**
- **3 medium unpeeled sweet potatoes, sliced very thin**
- **8 to 10 sheets phyllo pastry**
- **4 tbsp. melted butter or olive oil**
- **2 cups grated Gruyère cheese**
- **sea salt to taste**
- **freshly ground pepper to taste**

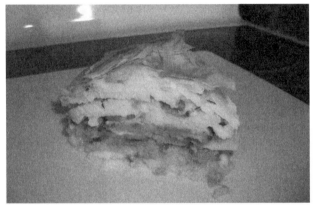

1. Preheat the oven to 350°F.

2. Mix the garlic, green onions, and rosemary in a small bowl and set aside.

3. Place the potatoes and sweet potatoes in a large pot and cover with water. Bring to a boil over high heat and cook for 5 to 8 minutes, or until tender. Drain and set aside to cool.

4. Place your phyllo sheets in a stack on a clean, dry surface. Cover them with a damp (not wet) cloth so they don't dry out. Have your melted butter or olive oil ready to brush onto your pastry sheets.

5. Brush the top sheet of phyllo lightly with butter and place it in the bottom of a lightly greased 10-inch springform pan (the edges should be hanging out of the pan). Do the same with the next piece of phyllo, but place it at a right angle to the first. Repeat these steps until you have 6 to 8 layers of phyllo and the base of your pan is covered.

6. Arrange one third of the potato and sweet potato slices on top of the phyllo crust, overlapping them slightly to form a single layer. Sprinkle with one third of the garlic, onion, and rosemary mix, and then one third of the grated Gruyère cheese. Season to taste with sea salt and pepper. Repeat until all of the potatoes, garlic mix, and cheese are used.

7. Gather the phyllo corners from around the edges of the pan and gently crumple them up and over the edges of the dish towards the middle of the pie. They will stay where you place them. Brush the phyllo corners with melted butter and crumple up two more pieces of phyllo to fill any gaps in the centre of the pie so it is completely covered.

8. Bake for 35 to 45 minutes, or until the crust is golden brown. Make sure you keep an eye on the pie as it bakes— if the phyllo browns too quickly, cover the pie with a piece of aluminum foil for the remainder of cooking.

9. Let stand for 10 minutes and then remove the ring of the springform pan carefully. Slice into wedges with a serrated knife. Serves 6 to 8.

Full of Beans and Lentils

If you can get beans or lentils into your diet once or twice a week, your body will be most grateful. The following chapter has my recipe for Baked Beans Sans Sugar *(page 115)*, where we use zesty spices and salsa instead of the traditional sugar and molasses. We also have instructions for how to make our Champion Veggie Burgers, *(page 122)* which don't fall apart and are very tasty.

Vegetarian Moussaka

vegetarian
gluten-free option

It takes a bit of work to make moussaka, but it is definitely worth the effort. You can also make it ahead of time and pop it in the oven before company arrives. When you make this dish for someone, they will know you think they are special.

If you have bell peppers or zucchini on hand, you can roast them with the eggplant and add them to the eggplant layer.

- **2 cups cooked chickpeas**
- **2 medium eggplants, cut into ¼-inch slices and salted***
- **2 to 3 large unpeeled potatoes, cut into ¼-inch slices**
- **1 tbsp. sunflower oil**
- **1 medium onion, chopped**
- **2 cloves garlic, minced**
- **1 (796 ml) can diced tomatoes, drained**
- **1 tbsp. dried oregano**
- **1 tbsp. dried basil**
- **½ tsp. ground cinnamon**
- **sea salt to taste**
- **freshly ground pepper to taste**
- **⅓ cup grated Parmesan cheese**
- **2 cups béchamel sauce** (page 69)**

1. Preheat the oven to 400°F.

2. Rinse the chickpeas, drain, and place in a medium-sized mixing bowl. Mash until the consistency resembles a coarse meal. Set aside.

3. Rinse the eggplant slices and pat them dry with paper towels. Place them about an inch apart on lightly greased baking sheets. Bake in the preheated oven for 15 minutes. Flip and bake for 10 minutes on the other side.

4. While the eggplants are baking, place the potatoes in a large pot and cover with water. Bring to a boil over high heat and cook for 10 minutes, or until soft. Drain and place in the bottom of a lightly greased 9" × 13" baking pan. Set aside.

5. Heat the oil in a Dutch oven over medium-high heat. Add the onion and garlic and sauté for 2 to 3 minutes, or until the onion is soft. Stir in the chickpeas, tomatoes, oregano, basil, cinnamon, salt, and pepper. Reduce the heat to low and simmer, uncovered, for 2 to 3 minutes, stirring occasionally. Set aside.

6. Preheat the oven to 350°F. Layer half the eggplant slices over the potatoes in the baking pan. Spread the chickpea mixture on top. Sprinkle with half the Parmesan cheese. Layer the remaining eggplant on top. Spread the béchamel sauce over the eggplant and sprinkle with the remaining Parmesan.

7. Bake for 30 minutes, or until golden brown. Let it sit for 5 to 8 minutes before serving. Serves 6 to 9.

*For detailed instructions on salting eggplants, see page 17.

**For the gluten-free option, use our gluten-free version of béchamel sauce from page 70.

Baked Beans Sans Sugar

vegan
gluten-free

Although I do love traditional baked beans with molasses, brown sugar, and maple syrup, I developed a sweet-free version for those who are watching their sugar intake. This one tastes just as good as the original, if not better. For more variety, use any combination of navy beans, black turtle beans, chickpeas, and red or white kidney beans.

- **3 cups navy beans, soaked overnight and rinsed**
- **2 medium onions, chopped**
- **3 unpeeled carrots, scrubbed and sliced**
- **2 cups diced celery**
- **3 to 4 cloves garlic, minced**
- **4 cups vegetable stock**
- **1 cup homemade salsa (page 68)**
- **1 to 2 chipotle or jalapeño peppers, minced (use gloves)**
- **2 tsp. smoked paprika**
- **2 tsp. dried oregano**
- **1 tsp. chili powder**
- **1 tbsp. Bragg Liquid Aminos**
- **1 tsp. sea salt**
- **1 tsp. freshly ground pepper**

1. Preheat the oven to 375°F.

2. Mix all of the ingredients in a large ovenproof pot or Dutch oven.

3. Bake, covered, in the preheated oven for 45 minutes. Reduce the heat to 250°F and bake for 5 to 6 hours, stirring occasionally. Add extra water if the mixture gets dry. The beans are done when you can squish a cooled bean between your tongue and the roof of your mouth.

4. Adjust the seasonings to your taste before serving. Serves 6.

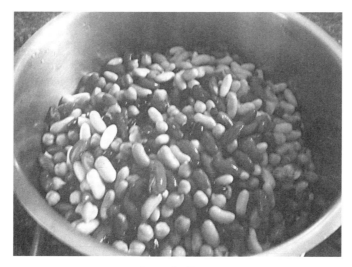

Pre-soaked beans

Mjadra (Lebanese Lentils, Rice, and Caramelized Onions)

vegan
gluten-free

This is a typical Middle Eastern recipe that works as a vegetarian main dish or a side dish. Try it with our Baked Lebanese-Spiced Kibbee (page 168) and/or Haida's Tabouli Salad (page 49).

- 1 cup uncooked brown or green lentils, rinsed
- 1 cup uncooked brown rice
- 2 cups water
- 1 bay leaf
- ½ tsp. ground cumin
- ½ tsp. cayenne pepper
- 1 (2-inch) piece cinnamon stick
- 1½ tsp. cumin seeds
- 1 tbsp. sunflower oil
- 2 large onions, sliced
- sea salt to taste
- freshly ground pepper to taste

1. Place the lentils, brown rice, water, bay leaf, ground cumin, cayenne, and cinnamon stick in a covered medium saucepan and bring to boil over high heat. Reduce the heat to low and simmer, without stirring, for 40 to 45 minutes, or until the lentils and rice are tender.

2. While the lentils and rice are cooking, heat a medium-sized, dry skillet over medium heat. Add the cumin seeds and cook, shaking the pan once in a while, until they darken a touch, about 1 minute. Add the oil and onions and sauté, stirring often, until the onions have caramelized, about 10 to 15 minutes. Stir in the sea salt and pepper.

3. Serve with the caramelized onions alongside the rice and lentil mixture. Serves 4 to 6.

Baked Falafels in Wraps

vegan

We served these falafels with a mix of chopped tomatoes, green onions, and parsley in wraps topped with tahini sauce.

- **3 cloves garlic**
- **6 green onions, sliced and divided**
- **3 cups cooked chickpeas, rinsed and drained**
- **2 tbsp. olive oil**
- **2 tsp. ground cumin**
- **2 tsp. ground coriander**
- **2 tsp. sea salt**
- **1 tsp. paprika**
- **1 tsp. ground turmeric**
- **¼ tsp. cayenne pepper**
- **1 tsp. baking soda**
- **½ cup chopped fresh parsley**
- **2 Roma tomatoes, diced**
- **8 whole wheat flour tortillas**
- **2 cups tahini sauce (page 70)**

1. Preheat the oven to 350°F.

2. Place the garlic in the bowl of a food processor and process until minced. Add 4 of the green onions and process to combine. Add the chickpeas and olive oil and pulse until evenly combined.

3. Add the cumin, coriander, salt, paprika, turmeric, cayenne, baking soda, and all but 2 tablespoons of the parsley. Pulse until the mixture is thick.

4. Drop the mixture by tablespoons onto a lightly greased baking sheet. Bake for 25 to 30 minutes, or until golden brown. Set aside.

5. In a small bowl, mix the remaining green onions and parsley with the diced tomatoes. Set aside.

6. Spread the wraps out on a work station. Put 2 falafel balls in each wrap, and then top with 1 tablespoon of tahini sauce and 1 tablespoon of the diced tomato and parsley mix. Roll up and serve with extra tahini sauce. Serves 4 to 6.

Zesty Beans, Rice, and Lentils

vegan
gluten-free

This colourful and nutrition-packed meal consists of black beans, brown rice, and green lentils with lots of great vegetables. Make it as zesty as you like by adding more or less jalapeño pepper and serve it with corn chips.

- 1 tbsp. sunflower oil
- 1 large onion, diced
- 1 green bell pepper, diced
- ¼ to 1 jalapeño pepper (depending on how spicy you want it to be), minced
- 3 cloves garlic, minced
- 1 cup uncooked green lentils, rinsed
- 1 cup uncooked brown rice
- ½ tsp. ground cumin
- 1 tsp. chili powder
- 1 tsp. dried oregano
- 3 cups water or vegetable stock
- 1 cup canned or frozen corn kernels
- 2 cups black beans, cooked, rinsed, and drained
- 1 cup homemade salsa (page 68) or store-bought salsa
- sea salt to taste
- freshly ground pepper to taste

1. Heat the oil in a large saucepan over medium-high heat. Add the onion and sauté for 2 to 3 minutes. Next add the green pepper, jalapeño pepper, and garlic and sauté for an additional 2 to 3 minutes, or until the vegetables soften.

2. Add the lentils, brown rice, cumin, chili powder, and oregano and mix to combine. Next add the water or stock and bring to a boil over high heat. Reduce the heat to low and simmer, covered, for 40 minutes without stirring.

3. Add the corn, black beans, salsa, salt, and pepper and cook until heated through. Serves 6.

Curried Chickpeas in Love

vegan
gluten-free

Curry and chickpeas is a match made in heaven. All you have to do is combine these "made for each other" ingredients and add some complementary food accessories, and you have a "happily ever after" story.

- 1 tbsp. sunflower oil
- 2 onions, minced
- 4 cloves garlic, minced
- 2 tsp. finely grated unpeeled fresh ginger
- 1 tsp. ground cinnamon
- 1 tsp. ground cumin
- 1 tsp. ground coriander
- sea salt to taste
- 1 tsp. cayenne pepper
- 1 tsp. ground turmeric
- 3 cups cooked chickpeas, rinsed and drained
- 1 (796 ml) can crushed tomatoes
- 1 cup chopped fresh cilantro, divided

1. Heat the oil in a large skillet over medium-high heat. Add the onions and sauté for 2 to 3 minutes, or until tender. Stir in the garlic, ginger, cinnamon, cumin, coriander, salt, cayenne, and turmeric. Reduce the heat to medium and cook for 1 minute, stirring constantly.

2. Mix in the chickpeas and tomatoes. Cover and continue to cook, stirring occasionally, until all the flavours are well blended, about 45 to 60 minutes. Remove from heat.

3. Stir in the cilantro just before serving, reserving 1 tablespoon for garnish. Serve with organic brown rice. Serves 4.

Black Bean and Mushroom Burritos

vegan

These burritos are delicious. You can serve them right away or freeze them for later. When reheating them from frozen, wrap them in tin foil and bake for 1 hour at 350°F.

- 1 tbsp. sunflower oil
- 1 onion, diced
- 3 cloves garlic, minced
- 1 green bell pepper, diced
- 1½ cups sliced button mushrooms
- 1 tsp. smoked paprika
- 1 tsp. chopped chipotle pepper or chipotle powder
- 1 tsp. ground cumin
- ½ tsp. sea salt
- ½ tsp. freshly ground pepper
- 3 cups cooked black beans, rinsed, drained, and lightly mashed
- 1½ cup homemade salsa (page 68) or store-bought salsa, plus extra for garnish
- ¼ cup chopped fresh cilantro
- 12 whole wheat tortillas
- vegan sour cream (page 67) for garnish

1. Preheat the oven to 350°F.

2. Heat the oil over medium heat in a large, heavy skillet. Add the onion and garlic and sauté for 2 to 3 minutes. Add the green pepper and mushrooms and sauté for an additional 2 to 3 minutes. Add the paprika, chipotle, cumin, sea salt, and pepper and sauté for another 1 to 2 minutes, or until all the vegetables are tender.

3. Mix in the beans and salsa and cook for 2 to 3 minutes, or until heated through. Adjust the seasonings to taste and mix in the cilantro. Remove from heat and set aside.

4. Spread the tortillas out over a clean, dry work surface. Divide the bean mixture evenly amongst them, spreading it in a line in the centre of each tortilla and leaving an inch on either side. Fold the short ends of each tortilla over the filling and hold them in place. Next fold one of the large ends over the filling and roll up, enclosing the filling. Place the rolled burritos in a lightly greased baking dish with the edge sides down.

5. Cover the dish with foil and bake for 20 to 25 minutes, or until the burritos are heated through. Garnish with more salsa and vegan sour cream if desired. Serves 4 to 6.

Red Lentil Dahl

vegan
gluten-free

One of the things I love about red lentils is that they fall apart into a smooth consistency after being cooked for a short time, which makes them perfect for dahl.

If you like some heat to your dahl, increase the amount of cayenne pepper used in this recipe.

- 1 tbsp. sunflower oil
- 1 large onion, diced
- 3 cloves garlic, minced
- 1 tbsp. grated fresh ginger
- 1 cup dried red lentils, rinsed
- 3 cups vegetable stock
- 1 (398 ml) can coconut milk
- 1 tsp. ground cumin
- 1 tsp. ground coriander
- 1 tsp. ground turmeric
- ¼ tsp. cardamom powder
- ¼ tsp. ground cinnamon
- ¼ tsp. cayenne pepper
- 1 tbsp. Bragg Liquid Aminos
- 1 (10 oz.) package frozen chopped spinach, thawed
- ¼ cup chopped fresh cilantro

1. Heat the oil in a large pot over medium-high heat. Add the onion, garlic, and ginger and cook, stirring often, for 3 to 4 minutes, or until the onions are translucent. Add the lentils, stock, coconut milk, cumin, coriander, turmeric, cardamom, cinnamon, cayenne, and Bragg's. Bring to a boil and then simmer over low heat for 25 to 30 minutes, or until the lentils are very tender.

2. Stir in the spinach and cook until heated through. Adjust the seasonings to taste and garnish with cilantro before serving. Serve with basmati rice and/or naan bread. Serves 4.

Champion Veggie Burgers

vegetarian with vegan option
gluten-free

It took much trial and error to finally come up with a good recipe for veggie burgers. I think you will like this one. If you want to make it vegan, just exchange the egg with a vegan egg replacement.

These burgers go great with our Nice Buns (page 183).

- **1 carrot, peeled and roughly chopped**
- **2 cloves garlic, minced**
- **2 cups cooked chickpeas, rinsed, drained, and towel-dried**
- **1 tsp. ground cumin**
- **1½ tsp. chili powder**
- **3 to 4 drops liquid smoke**
- **½ tsp. sea salt**
- **½ tsp. freshly ground pepper**
- **1 large egg**
- **3 tbsp. chickpea flour**
- **1 to 2 tbsp. sunflower oil**
- **1 tomato, sliced, for garnish**
- **6 whole lettuce leaves, washed and dried, for garnish**
- **Sweet Onion and Balsamic Relish (page 76) for garnish**

1. Place the carrot and garlic in the bowl of a food processor and pulse until the carrot is in small bits. Add the chickpeas, cumin, chili powder, liquid smoke, salt, and pepper and pulse to obtain a rough texture. Add the egg and chickpea flour and process briefly, until the contents are evenly mixed but coarse.

2. Heat the oil in a frying pan over medium-high heat. Divide the mixture into 6 even portions and form each portion into a patty with your hands. Fry the patties in batches for 2 to 3 minutes on each side, or until golden. Set the cooked patties on top of paper towel to drain while the remaining patties are being fried.

3. Serve the patties immediately, or let them cool and then grill them on the barbecue for extra flavour. Serve on a bun with lettuce, tomato, and sweet onion relish for garnish. Serves 4 to 6.

West Indian Lentil and Cheddar Rotis

vegetarian

A roti is a flatbread commonly used in the West Indies as a carrier for vegetables and curries. Rotis are also popular in India, where chapatis are used instead of tortillas.

- **2 cups dry green or brown lentils**
- **4 cups water**
- **2 sweet potatoes, peeled and cubed**
- **8 (8-inch) whole wheat tortillas or chapatis**
- **1 tbsp. sunflower oil**
- **1 large onion, chopped**
- **5 cloves garlic, minced**
- **1½ tbsp. grated unpeeled fresh ginger**
- **1 cup unpeeled, scrubbed, and diced carrots**
- **½ tsp. cumin seeds**
- **1½ tsp. sea salt**
- **2 tsp. curry powder**
- **1 tsp. ground coriander**
- **¼ tsp. cayenne pepper**
- **1 medium tomato, diced**
- **1 cup fresh or frozen peas**
- **2 cups grated cheddar cheese**
- **freshly ground pepper to taste**
- **plain yogurt for garnish**
- **mango or cilantro chutney for garnish**

1. Bring the lentils and water to a boil over high heat in a large covered saucepan. Reduce the heat to low and simmer, covered, for 20 minutes. Add the sweet potatoes and cook for an additional 10 minutes, or until the lentils and potatoes are tender. Set aside.

2. Preheat the oven to 350°F.

3. Place the tortillas or chapatis in a stack and wrap the stack in foil. Place the chapatis in the preheated oven to warm while preparing the rest of the ingredients.

4. Heat the oil in a large skillet over medium-high heat. Add the onion, garlic, ginger, carrots, and cumin seeds and sauté for 3 to 4 minutes, or until the onion is tender. Stir in the salt, curry powder, coriander, cayenne, tomato, peas, cheese, and the lentil-potato mixture. Reduce the heat to low and cook, uncovered, stirring occasionally, until heated through.

5. Remove the tortillas or chapatis from the oven and spread them out on a clean, dry work surface. Divide the filling evenly amongst the flatbread, spreading approximately 1 cup of the filling over half of each flatbread. Fold the flatbread over and garnish with yogurt and/or chutney. Serve immediately. Serves 4 to 6.

Lentil Torture (Oops! I mean Tourtière)

vegan

I make this dish at Christmas time for vegans and vegetarians. Making 1 or 2 tourtières is easy, but after making 15 or 20 of them in the Eat Well kitchen, I was calling them "Lentil Tortures." This is a great treat at anytime—you don't have to wait until Christmas.

- 1 tsp. sunflower oil
- 1 onion, chopped
- 2 stalks celery, diced
- 2 cloves garlic, minced
- 1 cup dried green or brown lentils, rinsed
- 2 unpeeled potatoes, diced
- 1½ tsp. ground cumin
- ½ tsp. ground cinnamon
- ½ tsp. dried thyme
- ½ tsp. dried sage

- ¼ tsp. ground cloves
- ¼ tsp. ground nutmeg
- ½ tsp. freshly ground pepper
- 1 tsp. sea salt, divided
- 3 cups water, divided
- 1 tbsp. Bragg Liquid Aminos
- 1 bay leaf
- 3 cups whole wheat flour
- ⅔ cup plus 1 tbsp. olive oil, divided

1. Heat the cooking oil in a large saucepan over medium heat. Add the onion and sauté 2 to 3 minutes. Add the celery and garlic and sauté for an additional 2 to 3 minutes, or until they are soft.

2. Increase the heat to high and stir in the lentils, potatoes, cumin, cinnamon, thyme, sage, cloves, nutmeg, pepper, and ½ teaspoon of the sea salt. Cook, stirring constantly, until heated through.

3. Add 2½ cups of the water, the Bragg's, and the bay leaf. Cover and let simmer over low heat for 25 minutes, or until the lentils are tender. Adjust the seasonings to taste, remove the bay leaf, and set aside to cool.

4. Preheat the oven to 350°F.

5. Combine the whole wheat flour with the remaining ½ teaspoon of salt in a large bowl. Slowly add ⅔ cup of the olive oil, mixing until a crumbly dough has formed.

6. Chill the remaining ½ cup of water until it is very cold and then add enough of the water to the dough to make it pliable but not sticky.

7. Place ⅔ of the dough between 2 sheets of wax paper and use a rolling pin to roll it into a circle about ¼ inch thick. Remove the wax paper and transfer the dough to the bottom of a 9-inch springform pan or a 10-inch pie plate. Press the dough into place in the pan, making sure no cracks or holes form in the dough as you do so, and leave the edges hanging over.

8. Pour the lentil and potato filling into the pie crust. Roll out the remaining ⅓ of the dough between 2 sheets of wax paper to form a circle about ¼ inch thick. Remove the wax paper and lay the dough circle on top of the filling, allowing the edges to hang over.

9. Fold and crimp the edges of the top and bottom halves of the crust together, and cut off any excess dough hanging over the edge of the pie plate. Pierce several holes in the top crust with a knife to release steam. Brush the top crust with the remaining 1 tablespoon of olive oil.

10. Bake in the preheated oven for 30 minutes, or until golden. Let stand for 5 to 10 minutes before serving. Serves 6 to 8.

Tip: If you have leftover dough, roll it out and cut out some shapes. Brush the bottom of the shapes with water and use them to decorate the top of the tourtière.

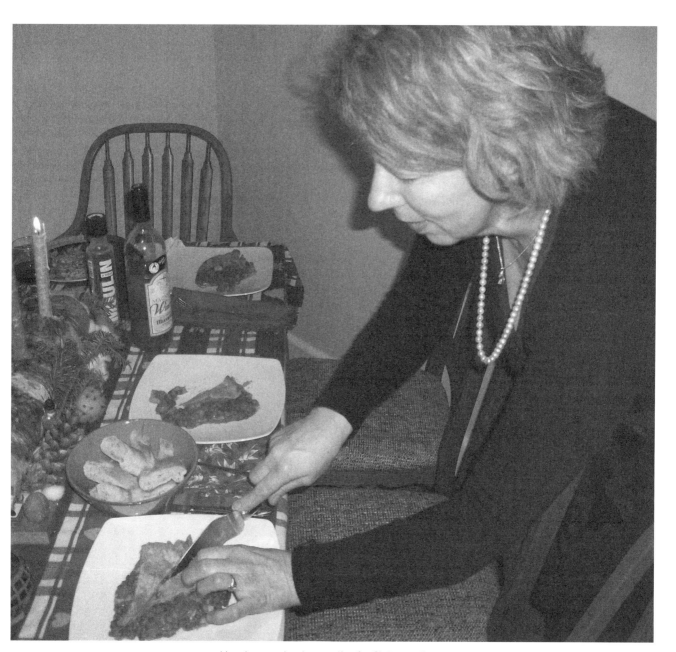

Here I am serving the tourtière for Christmas dinner.

Pastabilities

If you have the ingredients in your pantry, you can do up some very good company-worthy pasta meals quickly and easily. In this chapter, we included the recipes for our popular Roasted Vegetable Lasagna *(page 133)*, the West Indian–inspired Rasta Pasta *(page 128)* and a comfort food stand-by, Baked Three-Cheese Penne with Broccoli *(page 129)*.

Mouth-Watering Mediterranean Penne

vegetarian with vegan and non-vegetarian options

This recipe is very versatile—you can substitute the spinach for whatever vegetables are in season or whatever is in your fridge. Our customers always loved it when we used fiddleheads or asparagus in the early spring. Mushrooms, roasted bell peppers, and fresh diced tomatoes are other great options. If you want a little extra protein and you aren't cooking for a vegetarian or vegan, add some cooked sliced chicken. For the vegan option, omit the feta cheese.

- ½ cup pine nuts, slivered almonds, or other nuts
- 1 (450 g) package uncooked whole wheat penne
- 1 tbsp. sunflower oil
- 1 large red onion, sliced
- 3 cloves garlic, minced
- 6 to 8 sun-dried tomatoes, sliced
- 6 to 9 marinated artichokes*, sliced
- ½ cup olives* (any variety), pitted
- 4 cups fresh spinach or 2 cups any other fresh vegetable
- ¼ cup olive oil
- 2 tbsp. balsamic vinegar
- ½ cup crumbled feta cheese*
- 2 tbsp. thinly sliced fresh basil
- sea salt to taste
- freshly ground pepper to taste

1. Place the nuts in a large, dry skillet over medium-high heat. Cook, stirring constantly for 2 to 4 minutes, or until toasted and brown. Remove to a bowl and set aside.

2. Bring a large pot of water to a boil over medium-high heat. Add the penne and cook for 1 minute less than the directions on the package recommend. Drain, but don't rinse (rinsing removes the starch that helps the sauce adhere to the pasta). Set aside.

3. Heat the cooking oil in the skillet over medium-high heat. Add the onion and stir-fry for 2 minutes. Add the garlic, sun-dried tomatoes, artichokes, and olives. Stir-fry for an additional 2 to 3 minutes, or until the vegetables are soft.

4. Stir in the cooked pasta and the spinach or vegetables and sauté until the spinach wilts or the vegetables are slightly tender. Add the olive oil and balsamic vinegar and stir to coat. Stir in the feta cheese and fresh basil. Season well with sea salt and freshly ground pepper. Continue to cook, stirring constantly, until all ingredients are heated through. Serves 4 to 6.

*Optional

Rasta Pasta

vegan

This jazzy pasta dish is full of spicy West Indian flavours. I selected the most colourful vegetables for this recipe, but feel free to choose your own.

- **2 tbsp. sunflower oil, divided**
- **1 large onion, diced**
- **4 cloves garlic, minced**
- **4 tbsp. grated fresh ginger**
- **1 chili pepper, seeded and minced (wear gloves)**
- **4 cups diced pumpkin, squash, or sweet potato**
- **2 cups water or vegetable stock**
- **2 cups coconut milk**
- **2 tsp. ground coriander**
- **2 tsp. ground cumin**
- **1 tbsp. dried thyme**
- **1 tsp. white pepper**
- **½ tsp. grated fresh nutmeg**
- **½ tsp. ground allspice**
- **½ tsp. sea salt**
- **1 (450 g) package uncooked linguine or angel hair pasta**
- **1 red bell pepper, diced**
- **6 button mushrooms, chopped**
- **2 zucchinis, chopped**
- **½ cup fresh or frozen and thawed corn kernels**
- **1 cup broccoli florets, blanched**

1. Heat 1 tablespoon of the oil in a large skillet over medium heat. Add the onion, garlic, ginger, and chili pepper and sauté for 4 to 5 minutes. Stir in the pumpkin, squash, or sweet potato and the water or vegetable stock and cook, covered, for 15 to 20 minutes, or until the vegetables are tender.

2. Stir in the coconut milk, coriander, cumin, thyme, pepper, nutmeg, allspice, and salt and let simmer, uncovered, for 4 to 5 minutes. Using a hand blender, blend the contents of the skillet until smooth, or cool the mixture, place it in the bowl of a food processor, and process until smooth.

3. Place the sauce in a saucepan over low heat and keep warm while preparing the pasta and vegetables. Cook the pasta according to the directions on the package. Drain, but don't rinse. Set aside.

4. Heat the remaining tablespoon of oil in a large, clean skillet over medium-high heat. Add the red pepper, mushrooms, and zucchinis and sauté for 4 to 5 minutes. Stir in the corn and broccoli and sauté for 2 more minutes, or until the vegetables are tender.

5. Add the cooked pasta and sauce to the skillet and stir to combine. Bring the mixture to a simmer and cook until heated through. Serves 4 to 6.

Baked Three-Cheese Penne with Broccoli

vegetarian with non-vegetarian option

This baked pasta dish is as "comfort food" as they come. Looking for something a bit more exciting? Swap the Parmesan cheese for crumbled blue cheese. You can also add chunks of chicken, salmon, or tuna if you're looking for a meat option.

- 1 (450 g) package uncooked whole wheat penne
- 2 tbsp. butter
- 2 cloves garlic, minced
- 2 tbsp. unbleached white flour
- 2 cups milk
- ½ cup grated Parmesan cheese
- 2 cups grated cheddar cheese, divided
- ½ cup light cream cheese
- sea salt to taste
- freshly ground pepper to taste
- ½ tsp. grated fresh nutmeg
- 2 cups broccoli florets, blanched
- 1 tbsp. dried or chopped fresh parsley

1. Preheat the oven to 375°F.

2. Bring a large pot of water to a boil over medium-high heat. Add the penne to the water and cook for 1 minute less than the directions on the package recommend. Drain, but don't rinse (rinsing the pasta removes the starch that helps the sauce adhere to the pasta). Set aside.

3. In a large saucepan, melt the butter with the garlic over low heat. Remove the pan from the heat, add the flour, and stir it into the butter to form a thick, smooth paste. Add ½ cup of the milk and whisk until a smooth, white liquid has formed. Add the remaining 1½ cups of milk, the Parmesan cheese, 1 cup of the cheddar cheese, and the cream cheese and stir to combine.

4. Place the saucepan back onto the stove and turn the heat up to medium-high. Bring the sauce to a boil, stirring constantly. Once the sauce starts to boil and thicken, reduce the heat to low and simmer, stirring frequently, for 8 to 10 minutes, or until the consistency is like thick cream. Season with the sea salt, pepper and nutmeg.

5. Place the sauce, blanched broccoli, and cooked penne in a large bowl and stir to combine. Pour the mixture into a lightly greased 9" × 12" baking pan. Sprinkle with the remaining cheddar cheese and the parsley. Bake in the preheated oven for 35 to 45 minutes, or until the top is lightly browned. Serves 6

Pasta Puttanesca

vegan

This pasta dish was made by the Italian "ladies of the evening" because most of the ingredients were kept on hand and it was quick and easy to make. This recipe is just a guide, so look in your fridge and create your own version based on what you've got. If you have nuts or seeds, add them for extra protein.

- 1 (450 g) package uncooked spaghetti or angel hair pasta
- 1 tbsp. sunflower oil
- 1 large onion, sliced
- 2 cloves garlic, minced
- 1½ cups sliced mixed sweet bell peppers (the more colours, the prettier)
- 4 plum tomatoes, cut into wedges
- 4 anchovy filets, roughly chopped
- 1 tablespoon capers
- 12 black olives, pitted
- ½ tsp. chili flakes, or chili flakes to taste
- sea salt to taste
- freshly ground pepper to taste
- 1 to 2 tbsp. extra virgin olive oil
- finely chopped fresh parsley or basil for garnish

1. Bring a large pot of water to a boil over medium-high heat. Add the pasta to the water and cook for 1 minute less than the directions on the package recommend. Drain, but don't rinse (rinsing the pasta removes the starch that helps the sauce adhere to the pasta). Set aside.

2. Heat the oil in a large skillet over medium heat. Add the onion and garlic and sauté for 2 to 3 minutes. Stir in the bell peppers, tomatoes, anchovies, capers, olives, chili flakes, sea salt, pepper, and olive oil. Cook for 5 minutes, or until the vegetables are soft.

3. Add the cooked pasta to the skillet, allowing it to finish cooking in the sauce for another 2 to 3 minutes, or until the pasta is al dente and heated through.

4. Garnish with the parsley or basil and serve immediately. Serves 4 to 6.

Ligurian Bread and Garlic Pasta

vegetarian

This was a very popular choice in our catering business. It was also a favourite of the kitchen staff.

- **6 cloves garlic, peeled**
- **2 cups cubed fresh multigrain bread**
- **3 tbsp. red wine vinegar, divided**
- **¼ cup water**
- **½ tsp. sea salt**
- **½ tsp. freshly ground pepper**
- **¾ cup extra virgin olive oil**
- **1 cup chopped fresh parsley, divided**
- **2 cups uncooked penne pasta**
- **2 tomatoes, diced**
- **grated Parmesan cheese for garnish**

1. Place the garlic in the bowl of a food processor and process until minced. Add the bread, 2 tablespoons of the vinegar, and the water, and blend until combined. Mix in the salt and pepper. With the processor running, add the olive oil in a thin, steady stream. Next add all but 1 tablespoon of the parsley and blend to combine.

2. Place the pasta in a large pot of boiling salted water and cook for 8 to 10 minutes, or until the pasta is tender but firm. Drain, reserving ½ cup of the cooking liquid. Do not rinse.

3. While you are waiting for the pasta to cook, combine the tomatoes with the remaining tablespoons of parsley and vinegar in a medium-sized mixing bowl. Season with freshly ground pepper and set aside.

4. Replace the drained pasta in the pot and place over low heat. Pour the bread sauce over the pasta and stir until heated through, adding some of the reserved cooking liquid if the sauce is too thick. Garnish with the tomato mixture and Parmesan cheese. Serves 4.

Village Peppercorn Linguine

vegetarian

Green peppercorns are the unripened seeds of the Piper nigrum plant. They have a fresh flavour that is less pungent than black and white peppercorns and are often preserved in brine. They are used in cheeses, pâtés, and sauces and are an essential ingredient for making peppercorn steak.

- 1 (450 g) package uncooked linguine
- 1 tbsp. sunflower oil
- 2 large onions, sliced
- 12 to 14 medium-sized button mushrooms, sliced
- 1 tbsp. marinated green peppercorns
- 1 (250 g) package light cream cheese
- 1 (300 g) package frozen spinach, thawed and drained
- ½ tsp. sea salt
- ½ tsp. freshly ground pepper
- 1 large tomato, diced

1. Cook the linguine according to the directions on the package. Drain, reserving 1 cup of the cooking liquid. Do not rinse.

2. Heat the oil in a skillet over medium heat. Add the onions and cook for 5 to 7 minutes, or until lightly browned. Add the mushrooms and cook for 2 to 3 minutes more.

3. Squeeze the peppercorns between 2 spoons to squish them or chop them with a knife. Add them to the skillet along with the cream cheese, and stir until the cheese melts. Stir in the spinach, salt, and pepper.

4. Stir the cooked linguine into the mix and cook until all the ingredients are heated through. Add some of the reserved liquid if the sauce gets too thick during cooking. Garnish with the diced tomato before serving. Serves 4 to 6.

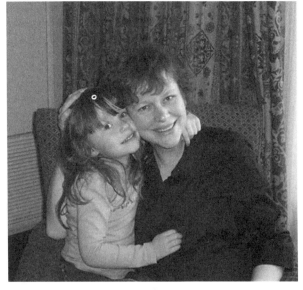

Lorenda with her daughter Taresa. I was so grateful when my friend Lorenda helped me out in the kitchen during the early Eat Well days. She taught me plenty and introduced me to this recipe, and it ended up being a regular in our repertoire right up until the end. Now it lives on.

Roasted Vegetable Lasagna

vegetarian

If I had a dollar for every lasagna I've made, I wouldn't have to write this cookbook. Needless to say, this lasagna was a bestseller.

- 1 red bell pepper, cut into 12 pieces
- 1 green bell pepper, cut into 12 pieces
- 1 large onion, cut into large chunks
- 1 zucchini, cut into ½-inch slices
- 10 to 12 mushrooms, halved
- 1 cup broccoli florets
- 1 cup cauliflower florets
- 2 tbsp. olive oil
- 1 tsp. dried oregano
- 1 tsp. dried basil
- 1 tsp. dried parsley
- 1 tsp. Bragg Liquid Aminos
- ½ tsp. freshly ground pepper
- 12 uncooked whole wheat lasagna noodles
- 1 (500g) container cottage cheese
- 1 cup grated Parmesan cheese, divided
- 4 cups Eat Well Tomato Sauce (page 67)
- 2 cups grated mozzarella cheese

1. Preheat the oven to 400°F.

2. Combine the red and green peppers, onion, zucchini, mushrooms, broccoli, and cauliflower in a large bowl. Drizzle with the olive oil and sprinkle with the oregano, basil, parsley, Bragg's, and pepper. Mix well.

3. Spread the vegetable mixture evenly over 2 lightly greased baking sheets, making sure the vegetables aren't crowded. Roast for 35 to 40 minutes, stirring and switching the placement of the sheets on the baking racks after 20 minutes.

4. While the vegetables are roasting, cook the lasagna noodles according to directions on the package. Drain, but don't rinse. Set aside.

5. When the vegetables have finished roasting, put them all back into the large bowl and mix with the cottage cheese and ½ cup of the Parmesan cheese.

6. Reduce the oven temperature to 375°F.

7. Lightly grease a 9" × 12" lasagna pan. Place 3 of the cooked lasagna noodles side by side, lengthwise, on the bottom of the pan. Cover the noodles with 1⅓ cups of the tomato sauce. Top with 3 more noodles and cover with another 1⅓ cups of the tomato sauce. Top with 3 more noodles and all of the vegetable mixture. Top the lasagna with the last 3 noodles and the remaining 1⅓ cups of the tomato sauce.

8. Sprinkle the mozzarella cheese and the remaining Parmesan cheese evenly over the top.

9. Place the lasagna in the preheated oven and bake for 35 to 45 minutes, or until the cheese is golden and bubbly and the lasagna is heated through. Let stand for 10 minutes before serving. Serves 6 to 8.

Italian Sausage or Beef Lasagna

This lasagna is easy to make, but full of all the flavours you love.

- **2 tbsp. olive oil**
- **2 lbs. Italian sausage meat or lean ground beef**
- **4 cups Eat Well Tomato Sauce (page 67)**
- **½ tsp. freshly ground pepper**
- **12 uncooked whole wheat lasagna noodles**
- **1 (500g) container cottage cheese**
- **½ cup dried parsley**
- **1 cup grated Parmesan cheese, divided**
- **2 cups shredded mozzarella cheese**
- **½ tsp. dried Italian seasoning**

1. Heat the oil in a large skillet over medium-high heat. Add the meat, break it up, and sauté, stirring constantly, until it is cooked through. Stir in the tomato sauce and simmer, uncovered, over low heat for 10 minutes. Set aside.

2. While the sauce is simmering, cook the lasagna noodles according to directions on the package. Drain, but don't rinse. Set aside.

3. In a medium-sized mixing bowl, combine the cottage cheese with the dried parsley and ½ cup of the Parmesan cheese. Set aside.

4. Preheat the oven to 350°F.

5. Lightly grease a 9" × 12" lasagna pan. Place 3 of the cooked lasagna noodles side by side, lengthwise, on the bottom of the pan. Cover the noodles with ⅓ of the meat sauce. Top with 3 more noodles and cover with another ⅓ of the meat sauce. Top again with 3 more noodles and the cottage cheese mixture. Top with the last 3 noodles and the remaining meat sauce.

6. In a clean medium-sized mixing bowl, combine the mozzarella cheese with the remaining ½ cup of the Parmesan cheese and the Italian seasoning. Sprinkle the cheese mixture evenly over the top of the lasagna.

7. Place the lasagna in the preheated oven and bake for 35 to 45 minutes, or until the cheese is nicely browned. Let stand for 10 minutes before serving. Serves 6 to 8.

Vegetable Tetrazzini

vegetarian with non-vegetarian option

For a Chicken Tetrazzini, add 3 to 4 cups of cooked chicken to the pasta and sauce mixture and substitute chicken stock for the vegetable stock.

- **1 (450 g) package uncooked spaghetti**
- **¼ cup butter**
- **10 to 12 button mushrooms, sliced**
- **2 carrots, peeled and sliced on the diagonal**
- **¼ cup all-purpose flour**
- **½ tsp. sea salt**
- **2 cups 1% milk**
- **1 cup vegetable stock**
- **1 cup of broccoli florets, blanched**
- **1 cup of cauliflower florets, blanched**
- **2 cups grated mozzarella cheese**
- **⅓ cup grated Parmesan cheese**
- **paprika to taste***

1. Preheat the oven to 425°F.

2. Cook the spaghetti according to the directions on the package. Drain, but do not rinse. Set aside.

3. While the spaghetti is cooking, melt the butter in a large skillet over medium heat. Add the mushrooms and carrots and sauté for 4 to 5 minutes. Add the flour and sea salt and stir until smooth. Add the milk and stock and cook, stirring constantly, for 5 minutes, or until the sauce has thickened to the consistency of cream. Add the broccoli, cauliflower, and cooked spaghetti and sauté until heated through.

4. Pour the mixture in a lightly greased baking dish. Top with the mozzarella and Parmesan cheeses and sprinkle with the paprika.

5. Bake for 25 to 30 minutes, or until hot and bubbly. Let stand for 10 minutes before serving. Serves 4 to 6.

*Optional

Pasta with Pumpkin Seed Pesto and Goat Cheese

vegetarian

There are some pretty strong flavours in this dish, but they complement one another rather than compete. Add your choice of sautéed vegetables to this recipe if you like.

- 1 (450 g) package uncooked angel hair pasta or spaghettini
- 5 to 6 tablespoons crumbled goat cheese
- 1 recipe Pumpkin Seed Pesto (page 78)
- 1½ cups cherry tomatoes, halved
- ½ tsp. sea salt
- ½ tsp. freshly ground pepper

1. Cook the pasta in a large pot according to directions on the package. Drain, but don't rinse.

2. Replace the hot pasta in the pot. Add the goat cheese and pesto and toss until the cheese is melted and the pesto coats the pasta. Add the tomatoes and any other sautéed vegetables you'd like to include. Cook over medium heat, stirring constantly, until heated through. Season with the sea salt and freshly ground pepper and serve immediately. Serves 4.

Chicken Choices

We have quite a variety of chicken choices for you in this chapter. Some are gluten-free, such as Chicken Zarzuela *(page 144)* or Chipotle-Roasted Chicken with Potatoes and Sweet Potatoes *(page 145)*. Some are dairy-free, including our Peruvian Roasted Chicken and Awesome Oven-Barbecued Chicken *(page 163)*. If you want something zesty, try the Tantalizing Thai Chicken Pot Pie *(page 149)* or "No Butter" Butter Chicken *(page 150)*. If you are seeking comfort food, the Scarborough Fair Corn Flake–Crusted Chicken *(page 147)* and Chicken Stew with Rosemary Dumplings *(page 155)* are both winners.

Chicken and Sausage Paella

dairy-free
gluten-free

The recipe calls for chicken and sausage, but you can add any protein you wish. Shrimp, salmon, mussels...the sky (or the sea) is the limit!

- **1½ cups chicken stock**
- **large pinch saffron**
- **2 tbsp. sunflower oil**
- **½ lb. Italian sausage, cut into ½-inch slices**
- **1 lb. boneless skinless chicken, cut into 1-inch squares**
- **1 onion, chopped**
- **1 green bell pepper, chopped**
- **3 cloves garlic, minced**
- **1½ cups uncooked brown rice**
- **1 (796 ml) can diced tomatoes**
- **1 tsp. ground turmeric**
- **1 tsp. smoked paprika or chipotle pepper**
- **sea salt to taste**
- **freshly ground pepper to taste**
- **1 cup frozen peas**
- **2 to 3 tbsp. chopped cilantro**

1. Heat the chicken stock in a medium saucepan over high heat until it comes to a boil. Add the saffron and set aside to steep.

2. While the saffron and stock are steeping, heat the oil in a skillet or wok over medium-high heat. Add the sausage and chicken and stir-fry for 3 to 4 minutes, or until browned. Stir in the onion, green pepper, and garlic and sauté for 5 minutes.

3. Stir in the rice, tomatoes, steeped chicken stock, turmeric, paprika or chipotle, salt, and pepper. Cover and bring to a boil. Simmer, covered, without stirring, for 40 minutes, or until the rice is tender.

4. Add the peas and cook for 4 to 5 more minutes, or until the peas are heated through. Adjust the seasonings to taste and garnish with the cilantro before serving. Serves 4 to 6.

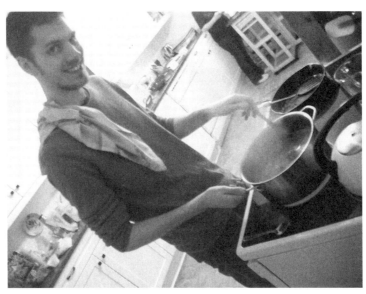

My awesome son Elliot also loves the kitchen. In this photo, he is helping me test recipes for this book.

Moroccan Chicken with Israeli Couscous

dairy-free

Israeli couscous—known in Hebrew as "ptitim"—is made of large, even-sized pearls of toasted pasta. You can find it in Middle Eastern grocery stores or upscale food markets.

- 1½ tsp. ground turmeric, divided
- 1½ tsp. ground cinnamon, divided
- ½ tsp. cayenne pepper
- 1 tsp. ground cumin
- 1 tsp. ground coriander
- 1 tsp. sea salt
- 1 tsp. freshly ground pepper
- 1 cup chickpea flour
- 3 tbsp. sunflower oil, divided
- 1 (3½ lb.) whole chicken, cut into pieces
- 2 onions, sliced
- 3 cloves garlic, minced
- 2½ cups chicken stock
- 2½ cups orange juice
- 2 cups Israeli couscous
- 3 tbsp. chopped fresh cilantro or parsley for garnish

1. Combine ½ teaspoon of the turmeric, ½ teaspoon of the cinnamon, and the cayenne, cumin, coriander, salt, and pepper in a medium-sized mixing bowl. Remove 3 teaspoons of spice mixture and set aside. Add the chickpea flour to the remaining seasonings and stir to combine.

2. Dredge the chicken pieces in the flour-spice mix and place on a plate.

3. Heat 2 tablespoons of the oil in a large pot over medium heat. Sauté the chicken in the oil in batches until browned, about 5 minutes per side. Remove from the pan.

4. Heat the remaining tablespoon of the oil in the pot. Add the onions and garlic and sauté for 5 minutes, or until browned. Add the remaining teaspoon of the turmeric and stir to combine. Next add the remaining reserved spice mix and the remaining teaspoon of cinnamon and mix well.

5. Stir in the chicken stock and orange juice. Add the chicken back into the pan and bring the liquid to a boil. Simmer, covered, over low heat for 45 minutes, or until the chicken is heated through and no longer pink inside.

6. Stir in the Israeli couscous and cook for another 10 to 12 minutes, or until the couscous is cooked al dente. Garnish with the fresh cilantro or parsley and serve immediately. Serves 4 to 6.

Moroccan Chicken with Israeli Couscous

Athena Chicken

gluten-free

Greek flavours abound in this tasty and tender chicken dish. Serve it with orzo or rice.

- **2 tbsp. olive oil**
- **1 (3½ lb.) whole chicken, cut into pieces**
- **6 garlic cloves, chopped**
- **1½ tsp. aniseed, crushed**
- **1 large fennel bulb*, sliced (retain the sprigs)**
- **1 (28 oz.) can diced tomatoes**
- **½ cup chicken stock**
- **1 tbsp. dried oregano, crumbled**
- **12 kalamata olives, pitted**
- **4 oz. feta cheese, crumbled**
- **sea salt to taste**
- **freshly ground pepper to taste**

1. Heat the olive oil in a large, heavy skillet over medium-high heat. Add the chicken pieces in batches if necessary and sauté until brown, about 5 minutes per side. Transfer the chicken to a plate.

2. Pour off all but 2 tablespoons of the drippings from the skillet and replace over heat. Add the garlic and aniseed to the drippings and stir-fry for 30 seconds. Next add the fennel and sauté for 4 to 5 minutes, or until soft. Stir in the tomatoes, stock, and oregano.

3. Return the chicken to the skillet and simmer over low heat, uncovered, for 25 minutes. Add the olives and cook, stirring occasionally, until the liquid has reduced to sauce consistency, about 6 to 8 minutes. Stir in the feta cheese and season to taste with the sea salt and freshly ground pepper. Garnish with some of the reserved fresh fennel sprigs. Serves 4 to 6.

*Fennel is a bulb that looks like a cross between an onion and celery, with fronds that look like dill. Fennel has a sweet, perfumey, anise-like flavour and imparts a light, bright, spring-like quality to foods. Fennel contains Vitamins A and C, as well as potassium and calcium.

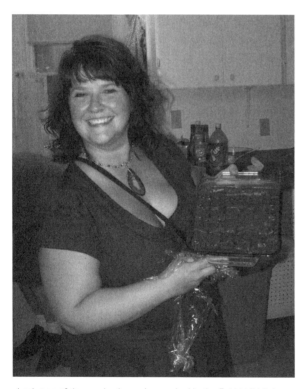

Lori, one of the magic elves who worked in the Eat Well kitchen. She loved to make this meal.

Chicken and Broccoli Crepes

To make a healthier crepe, we use 1% milk and whole wheat flour in this recipe.

- **3 cups plus 3 tbsp. 1% milk, divided**
- **2 eggs**
- **2 tbsp. butter, melted**
- **1 cup whole wheat flour**
- **¾ tsp. sea salt, divided**
- **3 tbsp. sunflower oil, divided**
- **2 lbs. boneless, skinless chicken breasts, cut into 1-inch cubes**
- **2 cups sliced mushrooms (any variety)**

- **1 tsp. dried basil or tarragon**
- **½ tsp. freshly ground pepper**
- **¼ tsp. grated fresh nutmeg**
- **1 tsp. Worcestershire sauce**
- **1 tsp. Bragg Liquid Aminos**
- **2 cups of fresh or frozen broccoli florets**
- **2 cups plus 2 tbsp. 1% milk**
- **2 tbsp. cornstarch**
- **2 tbsp. water**

1. In a small bowl, beat 1 cup plus 1 tablespoon of the milk with the eggs and butter. In a separate small bowl, combine the flour with ¼ teaspoon of the salt. Add the flour mixture to the egg mixture and beat until smooth. Cover and refrigerate the batter for 1 hour or overnight.

2. In a large saucepan, heat 1 tablespoon of the oil over medium heat. Add half of the chicken pieces and stir to keep them from sticking. Cook, stirring often, for 4 to 6 minutes, or until browned. Remove to a plate. Add another tablespoon of oil to the saucepan and stir-fry the remainder of the chicken until browned.

3. Return the reserved cooked chicken back to the pan. Stir in the mushrooms, broccoli (if using fresh broccoli), basil or tarragon, pepper, Worcestershire sauce, and the remaining ½ teaspoon of salt and cook for 3 to 4 minutes. Set aside.

4. Make a slurry by mixing the cornstarch and the water in a small bowl. Set aside.

5. Stir 2 cups of the remaining milk and the frozen broccoli (if using frozen) into the chicken mixture. Bring to a boil, stirring constantly. Re-stir the slurry and then slowly add it to the mixture. Keep stirring until the sauce becomes thick and bubbly. Remove the pan from the heat and set aside.

6. Preheat the oven to 250°F.

7. Heat the remaining tablespoon of oil in a lightly greased 9-inch skillet over medium-high heat. Re-stir the chilled crepe batter and pour approximately ¼ cup into the centre of skillet. Lift and tilt pan to coat the bottom evenly with the batter. Place the pan back over the heat and cook for 1 to 2 minutes, or until the top of the batter appears dry. Flip the crepe and cook for 15 to 20 seconds longer. (It is usually a rule that the first crepe never turns out, so don't despair if your crepe doesn't look how you expected—keep trying!)

8. Remove the crepe to an ovenproof plate and keep warm in the preheated oven. Repeat the cooking steps with the remaining crepe batter, greasing the skillet as needed. Makes about 10 crepes.

9. When all the crepes are cooked, reheat the chicken-broccoli mixture over medium heat. Place 1 warm crepe on a plate. Pour about ¼ cup of the chicken and broccoli mixture in a line in the middle of the crepe, leaving two inches on either side. Fold the short sides of the crepe in, then fold one of the larger sides over and roll. Set aside on a serving plate. Repeat the filling and rolling steps with the remaining crepes. Serve 2 crepes per person. Serves 4.

Balsamic Chicken with Bosc Pears

dairy-free
gluten-free

I am a big fan of balsamic vinegar so I'll try it with almost anything. This recipe is a success! We served this with jasmine rice.

- **1 to 2 tbsp. sunflower oil**
- **3 Bosc pears, peeled, cored, and cut into wedges**
- **4 boneless, skinless chicken breasts**
- **1 cup chicken stock**
- **3 tbsp. balsamic vinegar**
- **2 tbsp. cornstarch**
- **2 tbsp. water**

1. Heat 1 tablespoon of the oil in a large skillet over medium heat. Add the pear wedges and sauté for 2 to 3 minutes, or until lightly browned and tender. Transfer to a plate.

2. If needed, add the remaining tablespoon of oil to the skillet. Place the chicken breasts in the pan and cook for 3 to 4 minutes per side, or until brown on each side.

3. Add the chicken stock and balsamic vinegar and bring to a boil. Simmer, covered, over low heat for 15 to 20 minutes, or until the chicken feels firm and juices run clear.

4. In a small bowl, make a slurry by combining the cornstarch with the water. Add it to the skillet, stirring constantly until the sauce has thickened.

5. Return the pears to the skillet and cook for another 2 to 3 minutes, or until heated through. Serves 4

Herb-Roasted Chicken and Vegetables

In this dish, stuffing the chicken with fresh herbs infuses it with flavour, while the high oven temperature yields a crispy skin and juicy chicken.

- **2 unpeeled carrots, scrubbed and cut into 2-inch chunks**
- **1 lb. unpeeled fingerling potatoes or 4 medium potatoes, washed and cut into 2-inch chunks**
- **1 onion, roughly chopped**
- **2 leeks, halved lengthwise and then crosswise (white and light-green parts only)**
- **10 cloves garlic, peeled, plus 2 cloves garlic, minced**
- **¼ cup plus 2 tablespoons olive oil, divided**
- **1 tbsp. Bragg Liquid Aminos**
- **2½ tsp. freshly ground pepper, divided**
- **½ tsp. dry rosemary or 1 tsp. fresh rosemary**
- **1 (4-5 lb.) whole chicken**
- **1½ tbsp. salt**
- **1 tbsp. dry or fresh thyme**
- **½ tbsp. dry or fresh sage**
- **2 tbsp. chopped fresh parsley**
- **1 cup white wine**

1. Place the carrots, potatoes, onion, leeks, and the 10 whole cloves of garlic in a large bowl and toss to combine. Drizzle the vegetables with ¼ cup of the olive oil and the Bragg's and sprinkle with the rosemary and ½ teaspoon of the pepper. Toss to coat. Place the vegetables in a roasting pan and set aside.

2. Preheat the oven to 450°F.

3. Wash the chicken and pat it dry. Season the inside and outside with the salt and the remaining 2 teaspoons of pepper.

4. In a small bowl, combine the remaining 2 cloves of minced garlic with the thyme, sage, parsley, and the remaining 2 tablespoons of olive oil. Pour the garlic mixture over the chicken and rub it evenly over the outside and in the cavity. Place the chicken on top of the vegetables in the roasting pan. Place some of the vegetables in the cavity of the chicken if desired.

5. Place the roasting pan into the preheated oven and roast for about 1 hour. Remove and pour the white wine over the chicken. Replace in the oven roast for another 30 minutes, or until the chicken is golden brown and the juices run clear.

6. Move the chicken onto a platter and let it stand for 10 minutes before carving. Cut the chicken into pieces. Serve with the pan juice and roasted vegetables. Serves 4 to 6.

Chicken Zarzuela

gluten-free
dairy-free

This Spanish dish reminds me of Don Ross, guitar player extraordinaire! He plays a terrific piece called "Zarzuela." I believe this dish tastes as yummy as his piece sounds. This is delicious served with either potatoes or rice.

- **2 tbsp. sunflower oil, divided**
- **16 skinless chicken thighs**
- **½ cup dry white wine**
- **2 Spanish onions, chopped**
- **6 cloves garlic, minced**
- **1 (796 ml) can diced tomatoes**
- **½ cup chicken stock**
- **4 tsp. sweet paprika**
- **1 tsp. dried oregano**
- **1 tsp. sea salt**
- **½ tsp. freshly ground pepper**
- **large pinch saffron**
- **2 tbsp. hot water**
- **½ cup ground almonds**
- **1 tbsp. lemon juice**
- **1 cup green olives, pitted and halved**
- **¼ cup chopped fresh parsley for garnish**

1. Preheat the oven to 375°F.

2. Heat 1 tablespoon of the oil in a large skillet over medium-high heat. Add the chicken thighs in batches and cook for 2 to 3 minutes per side, or until browned on each side. Transfer the cooked chicken pieces to a 9" × 13" glass baking dish.

3. Add the wine to the skillet and bring to a boil, stirring to scrape up the brown bits from the bottom of the pan. Pour over the chicken.

4. Warm the remaining tablespoon of oil in the skillet. Add the onions and garlic and sauté until golden, about 4 minutes. Stir in the tomatoes, stock, paprika, oregano, sea salt, and pepper. Bring to a boil and pour over the chicken.

5. Cover the baking dish loosely with foil and bake in the preheated oven for about 40 minutes, or until the chicken is no longer pink inside.

6. While the chicken is baking, crumble the saffron into a small mixing bowl. Pour in the hot water and let sit for 5 minutes. Stir in the ground almonds and lemon juice.

7. When the chicken is no longer pink inside, remove the baking dish from the oven and stir in the olives and the saffron and almond mixture. Remove the foil and replace in the oven. Bake, uncovered, for another 10 minutes. Garnish with the parsley before serving. Serves 6 to 8.

Chipotle-Roasted Chicken with Potatoes and Sweet Potatoes

gluten-free
dairy-free

Chipotles are smoked jalapeño peppers that add a lovely "sweet with heat" flavour to your meal. You can find them by the can in the Mexican section of your grocery store or in ground powder form in the spice aisle.

- **1 whole chipotle pepper, minced, or 2 tsp. ground chipotle pepper**
- **1½ tsp. paprika**
- **1 tsp. ground cumin**
- **1½ tsp. dried oregano**
- **2 unpeeled sweet potatoes, washed and cut into wedges**
- **1½ lbs. small unpeeled potatoes, washed and cut into wedges**
- **1 tbsp. sunflower oil**
- **2 tsp. brown sugar**
- **1 (3 lbs.) whole chicken, cut into pieces**
- **2 tsp. chopped fresh cilantro**

1. Preheat the oven to 400°F.

2. Combine the chipotle pepper, paprika, cumin, and oregano in a small mixing bowl.

3. In a separate large bowl, toss the sweet potatoes and potatoes with the oil and 1 tablespoon of the spice mixture.

4. Add the brown sugar to the remaining spice mixture and stir to combine. Rub the chicken pieces with the remaining spice mixture so that each piece is evenly coated.

5. Arrange the chicken pieces on one half of a lightly greased baking sheet. Arrange the potatoes and sweet potatoes in a single layer on the other half of the pan. Loosely cover the chicken and potatoes with aluminum foil.

6. Bake in the preheated oven for 40 minutes. Remove the foil, turn and rearrange the potatoes, and return to the oven. Bake, uncovered, for 20 minutes longer, or until the chicken juices run clear and the potatoes are tender. Garnish with the cilantro before serving. Serves 4.

Ginger-Cashew Chicken

gluten-free
dairy-free

This dish was very popular in the Eat Well kitchen. We served this with scented jasmine rice.

You can buy pickled ginger at any Asian grocery store.

- **2 tsp. cornstarch**
- **1½ cups chicken stock**
- **2 tbsp. Bragg Liquid Aminos**
- **2 tbsp. pickled ginger juice (if you have it)**
- **1½ cups cashews for garnish**
- **1 to 2 tbsp. oil**
- **4 boneless, skinless chicken breasts, sliced into strips**
- **1 large onion, sliced**
- **1 tbsp. grated fresh unpeeled ginger**
- **2 cloves garlic, minced**
- **4 cups broccoli florets**
- **2 medium carrots, sliced**
- **⅓ cup pickled ginger slices, sliced into strips, for garnish**

1. In a medium-sized mixing bowl, combine the cornstarch, chicken stock, Bragg's, and pickled ginger juice, stirring until smooth. Set aside.

2. Place the cashews in a large, dry skillet over medium-high heat. Cook, stirring constantly and watching carefully, for 3 to 4 minutes, or until toasted and brown. Remove to a bowl.

3. Heat 1 tablespoon of the oil in the skillet over medium-high heat. Add the chicken in batches and stir-fry for 7 to 9 minutes, or until browned and cooked through. Remove the cooked chicken to a plate.

4. Heat another tablespoon of oil in the skillet if needed. Add the onion, fresh ginger, and garlic and stir-fry for 3 minutes. Add the carrots and sauté for another 2 to 3 minutes. Add the broccoli and stir-fry until the vegetables are tender but crisp.

5. Return the chicken to the skillet. Re-stir the cornstarch mixture and pour it over the chicken and vegetables. Cook, stirring constantly, until the mixture boils and thickens, about 2 minutes.

6. Garnish with the pickled ginger and toasted cashews. Serve with rice, if desired. Serves 4 to 6.

Scarborough Fair
Corn Flake-Crusted Chicken

Simon and Garfunkel knew what they were singing about when they combined these great herbs: parsley, sage, rosemary, and thyme. You will enjoy these seasonings in our healthy version of oven-baked chicken. A little singing can make this meal taste much better.

Serve this with our Oven Potato or Sweet Potato Fries (page 63).

- **3 cups corn flakes**
- **1 tsp. dried parsley**
- **1 tsp. dried sage**
- **1 tsp. dried rosemary**
- **1 tsp. dried thyme**
- **sea salt to taste**
- **freshly ground pepper to taste**
- **½ cup buttermilk**
- **½ tsp. cayenne pepper**
- **4 boneless, skinless chicken breasts (sliced in half if large)**

1. Preheat the oven to 400°F

2. Place the cornflakes, parsley, sage, rosemary, thyme, sea salt, and pepper in the bowl of a food processor. Pulse until the flakes are coarsely chopped. Transfer to a wide mixing bowl.

3. In another wide bowl, mix the buttermilk with the cayenne pepper. Dip the chicken breasts into the buttermilk mixture and then roll in the cornflake crumb mixture to coat. Place the breaded chicken breasts on a lightly greased baking sheet.

4. Bake in the preheated oven for 35 to 45 minutes, or until the chicken has browned and the juices run clear. Serves 4.

Garam Masala and Cashew Chicken

gluten-free
dairy-free

This flavourful chicken and vegetable dish can be served with basmati rice and/or naan bread.

- **2 to 3 tbsp. sunflower oil**
- **4 boneless, skinless chicken breasts, sliced into 2-inch cubes**
- **1 onion, diced**
- **2 cloves garlic, minced**
- **2 tsp. minced fresh unpeeled ginger**
- **1 tbsp. minced seeded jalapeño pepper***
- **2 tbsp. garam masala (page 18)**
- **1 (10 oz.) package frozen chopped spinach, thawed and drained**
- **1 cup chicken stock**
- **1 tbsp. Bragg Liquid Aminos**
- **1 cup chopped toasted cashews for garnish**
- **3 tbsp. chopped fresh cilantro for garnish**

1. Heat 2 tablespoons of the oil in a deep skillet over medium-high heat. Add the chicken cubes and stir-fry for 3 to 4 minutes, or until browned. Transfer the cooked chicken to a plate.

2. Add the onion, garlic, and ginger to skillet, along with an additional tablespoon of oil if needed. Cook, stirring occasionally, for 3 minutes. Add the jalapeño pepper and garam masala and cook, stirring constantly, for 1 minute. Stir in the spinach, stock, and Bragg's.

3. Return the chicken to the skillet and cook, covered, over medium-high heat for 20 to 25 minutes, or until the juices run clear. Adjust the seasonings to taste and garnish with the cashews and cilantro before serving. Serves 4.

*Optional

Tantalizing Thai Chicken Pot Pie

gluten-free
dairy-free

Would you like a little excitement and heat in your life? This recipe is a wonderful symphony of Thai flavours—one that will impress your friends at a dinner party.

- 1½ cups uncooked organic brown rice
- 4 cups plus 4 tablespoons water, divided
- 3 large sweet potatoes, peeled and cubed
- 2 white potatoes, peeled and cubed
- 1 (398 ml) can coconut milk, divided
- 3 tbsp. chopped fresh cilantro, divided
- 1 lime, zest and juice, divided
- 1 to 2 tbsp. sunflower oil
- 4 boneless, skinless chicken breasts, sliced into 2-inch cubes

- 1 red bell pepper, cut into 2-inch strips
- 1 green bell pepper, cut into 2-inch strips
- 3 unpeeled carrots, scrubbed and grated
- 1 (thumb-sized) piece unpeeled fresh ginger, grated
- 3 cloves garlic, minced
- 1 tbsp. your choice of curry paste
- 1 tbsp. **Bragg Liquid Aminos**
- 2 tbsp. cornstarch

1. Place the rice and 4 cups of the water in a medium saucepan. Bring to a boil over high heat. Reduce the heat to low and simmer, covered, for 45 minutes, or until tender.

2. While the rice is cooking, place the sweet and white potatoes in a large pot and cover with water. Bring to a boil over high heat. Reduce the heat to medium and cook until the potatoes are soft. Drain the potatoes and mash them with 2 tablespoons of the coconut milk, 1 tablespoon of the chopped cilantro, and ½ teaspoon of the lime juice. Set aside.

3. Heat 1 tablespoon of the oil in a large skillet over medium-high heat. Add half the chicken pieces and stir-fry for 2 to 3 minutes, or until browned. Transfer the cooked chicken pieces to a plate. Repeat the previous steps with the remaining uncooked chicken.

4. Heat the remaining tablespoon of oil if needed. Add the red and green peppers and stir-fry for 2 minutes. Next add the grated carrots, ginger, and garlic and sauté for an additional 2 minutes.

5. Return the chicken to the skillet. Stir in the curry paste and Bragg's and the remaining lime zest and juice and coconut milk and bring to a boil. Reduce the heat to low and simmer, covered, for 20 minutes.

6. Make a slurry by combining the cornstarch with the remaining 4 tablespoons of water in a small mixing bowl. Stir the slurry into the chicken mixture and keep cooking for a minute, or until the sauce has thickened. Stir in the remaining cilantro and set aside.

7. Preheat the oven to 350°F.

8. Remove the cooked rice from the pot and press it into the bottom of a lightly greased 9" × 11" baking dish. Pour the chicken mixture on top of the rice, then top with the mashed potato mix.

9. Bake in the preheated oven for 35 to 45 minutes, or until the potatoes are firm. Let stand for 5 minutes before serving. Serves 6.

"No Butter" Butter Chicken

gluten-free

Traditional butter chicken is loaded with cream and butter. Our ingredients are easier to live with, and may allow you to live longer. We serve this dish with brown basmati rice.

- **1 to 2 tbsp. olive oil**
- **1 (3 lb.) whole chicken, cut into pieces and skin removed**
- **2 onions, diced**
- **5 cloves garlic, minced**
- **2 tbsp. grated fresh unpeeled ginger**
- **2 tsp. chili powder**
- **1 tsp. ground turmeric**
- **1 (6-inch) cinnamon stick or 1 tsp. ground cinnamon**
- **1 (796 ml) can diced tomatoes**
- **1 tbsp. brown sugar**
- **½ tsp. sea salt**
- **½ tsp. freshly ground pepper**
- **1 cup fat-free yogurt or sour cream**
- **¼ cup chopped fresh cilantro**

1. Heat the oil in a large, deep skillet over medium-high heat. Add the chicken pieces in batches so as not to crowd the pan and sauté for 5 to 6 minutes, or until browned. Transfer the cooked chicken to a plate.

2. Heat another tablespoon of oil in the skillet if needed. Add the onions and garlic and sauté, stirring often, until tender, about 4 to 5 minutes. Stir in the ginger, chili powder, turmeric, and cinnamon, and sauté for 1 additional minute. Stir in the tomatoes, brown sugar, salt, and pepper.

3. Add the reserved chicken and simmer, uncovered, over low heat for 25 to 30 minutes, stirring occasionally. Remove about 1 cup of the sauce and pour it into a medium-sized mixing bowl. Stir in the yogurt or sour cream. Stir the yogurt sauce into the chicken mixture and cook until heated through. Garnish with the cilantro. Serves 4 to 6.

40 Cloves of Garlic Chicken

gluten-free
dairy-free

Don't let the number 40 scare you. The longer the garlic cooks, the sweeter and milder it becomes.

- 1 (3 lb.) whole chicken, cut into pieces and skin removed
- 1 tbsp. olive oil
- 40 cloves of garlic, peeled*
- 10 shallots, peeled
- ½ cup white wine
- ½ tsp. sea salt
- ½ tsp. freshly ground pepper
- 1 tbsp. chopped fresh rosemary or 1 tsp. dried rosemary
- 1½ cups chicken stock
- 2 tbsp. chopped chives or green onions for garnish

1. Heat the oil in a large, deep skillet over medium heat. Add the chicken pieces in batches so as not to crowd the pan and sauté each batch for 4 to 5 minutes, or until browned.

2. Add the garlic and shallots. Shake the pan to move the garlic and shallots under the chicken pieces. Cook for 10 to 15 minutes, or until the garlic and shallots brown lightly.

3. Pour the wine into the pan while scraping the bottom to release the brown bits. Stir in the salt, pepper, rosemary, and stock and bring to a boil. Reduce the heat to low, cover, and simmer gently for 30 to 35 minutes, or until the chicken juices run clear.

4. Garnish with the chives or green onions before serving. Serves 6.

*This is the easiest way to peel garlic without mess: Take your garlic bulbs and hit them on the counter to separate the cloves. Place all the cloves into a metal bowl and cover it with another metal bowl. Then shake the dickens out of it. Presto! You have peeled garlic.

Georgia's Malaysian Chicken and Sweet Potato Curry

gluten-free
dairy-free

We were very lucky to have Georgia, who has lived and travelled all over the world (including Malaysia), working in our kitchen for a couple of years. She introduced us to this very tasty and pretty dish and now I'm introducing it to you. We served this with jasmine rice and stir-fried snow peas.

- 1 large onion, chopped
- 5 cloves garlic, peeled
- 1 (thumb-sized) piece fresh unpeeled ginger, sliced
- 5 tbsp. curry powder
- ½ tsp. cayenne pepper
- 1 tbsp. Bragg Liquid Aminos
- 1 tbsp. sunflower oil
- 4 boneless, skinless chicken breasts, sliced into 2-inch cubes
- 1 (398 ml) can coconut milk
- 1 cup chicken stock
- 2 to 3 sweet potatoes, peeled and cut into 1-inch cubes
- 3 tbsp. chopped fresh cilantro

1. Place the onion, garlic, and ginger in the bowl of a food processor and process until puréed. Add the curry powder, cayenne, and Bragg's and process to form a thick paste. Mix in a little water if the mixture is too thick.

2. Heat the oil in a wok or large, deep skillet over medium heat. Add the onion and curry mixture and stir-fry for 1 to 2 minutes, or until it is fragrant and toasted.

3. Increase the heat to medium-high and add the chicken cubes. Cook, stirring constantly, for 3 to 4 minutes, or until browned. Add the coconut milk, chicken stock, and sweet potatoes and bring to a boil. Decrease the heat to low and simmer, covered, for 20 to 25 minutes, or until the sweet potatoes are tender.

4. Adjust the seasonings to taste and garnish with the cilantro before serving. Serves 4

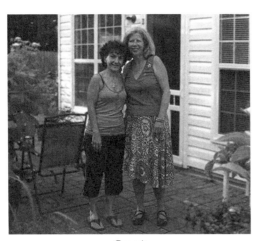

Georgia

Sweet potatoes are an excellent food source. They are low in sodium, and very low in saturated fat and cholesterol. They are also a good source of dietary fiber, vitamin B6 and potassium, and a very good source of vitamin A, vitamin C, and manganese. And they taste yummy!

Indonesian Orange and Peanut Chicken

gluten-free
dairy-free

If you want to impress your friends without a lot of preparation or a lot of work, they will be none the wiser with this very simple recipe.

- ½ **cup flaked coconut**
- **2 tbsp. peanuts**
- **3 tbsp. crunchy-style peanut butter**
- ½ **cup orange juice**
- **2 tbsp. curry powder**
- ½ **cup water**
- **1 tbsp. Bragg Liquid Aminos**
- **4 boneless, skinless chicken breasts**
- **1 red bell pepper, sliced**
- **1 green bell pepper, sliced**

1. Preheat the oven to 350°F.

2. Place the coconut and peanuts in a dry skillet over medium heat and cook, stirring constantly, until lightly toasted. Be careful they don't overcook. Set aside to cool.

3. Blend the peanut butter, orange juice, curry powder, water, and Bragg's together in a medium-sized mixing bowl to form pourable liquid. Add extra water if the consistency is too thick.

4. Pour 3 to 4 tablespoons of the sauce into the bottom of a lightly greased baking pan. Place the chicken breasts on top of the sauce, and then pour the remaining sauce on top. . Arrange the red and green peppers on the chicken. Sprinkle the toasted coconut and peanuts over the peppers.

5. Bake in the preheated oven for 50 minutes, or until the chicken is firm and the juices run clear. Serve with rice or noodles. Serves 4.

Persian Honey-Spiced Chicken

gluten-free
dairy-free

Here is an interesting and exotic way to enjoy chicken and to impress your family or guests. You can also substitute the chicken for tofu.

- **1 lemon, zest and juice**
- **¼ cup olive oil**
- **½ tsp. sea salt**
- **½ tsp. freshly ground pepper**
- **1 tsp. dried oregano**
- **2 cloves garlic, minced**
- **4 boneless, skinless chicken breasts or 6 boneless, skinless chicken thighs, cut into pieces the size of a deck of cards**
- **¼ cup honey**
- **½ recipe of Dukkah (page 28)**

1. Combine the lemon zest and juice, olive oil, salt, pepper, oregano, and garlic in a medium-sized mixing bowl.

2. Place the chicken pieces in the marinade, making sure all pieces are coated. Let stand for half an hour or more.

3. Preheat the barbecue or grill to medium-high heat or turn on the oven broiler and adjust the oven rack to 6 inches from the element.

4. Barbecue, grill, or broil the chicken for 5 to 7 minutes on each side, or until it is firm and the juices run clear.

5. Drizzle the cooked chicken pieces with a small amount of the honey and sprinkle them with the dukkah before serving. Serves 4 to 6.

Chicken Stew with Rosemary Dumplings

Juicy chunks of chicken and vegetables in a thick, savoury sauce topped off with light rosemary dumplings make this the ultimate comfort food. This meal always sold out quickly from the Eat Well kitchen.

- **5 cups chicken stock**
- **2 to 3 lbs. skinned chicken thighs and drumsticks**
- **1 cup plus 3 tbsp. unbleached white flour, divided**
- **½ cup whole wheat flour**
- **1 tbsp. plus ½ tsp. chopped fresh or dry rosemary**
- **2 tsp. baking powder**
- **¾ tsp. sea salt, divided**
- **2 tbsp. cold butter**
- **½ cup skimmed milk**
- **1 tbsp. sunflower oil**
- **1½ cups sliced celery**
- **1 large onion, sliced**
- **3 small unpeeled carrots, scrubbed and sliced**
- **1 cup halved button mushrooms**
- **½ tsp. dried or fresh thyme**
- **½ tsp. dried or fresh sage**
- **¼ tsp. freshly ground pepper**
- **2 unpeeled potatoes, washed and cubed**

1. In a large pot, bring the chicken stock to boil over medium-high heat. Reduce the heat to medium-low, add the chicken, cover, and simmer for 30 minutes, or until the meat falls off the bones easily.

2. While the chicken is cooking, whisk together 1 cup of the white flour, the whole wheat flour, 1 tablespoon of the rosemary, the baking powder, and ½ teaspoon of the salt in a medium-sized mixing bowl. Using a pastry blender or 2 knives, cut in the butter until the mixture resembles coarse crumbs. Using a fork, slowly stir in enough of the milk to transform the mixture into a sticky dough. Set aside.

3. When the chicken is cooked, transfer the meat to a plate using a slotted spoon, reserving the stock liquid. Allow the chicken to cool, then remove the meat from the bones and cut it into bite-size chunks.

4. Heat the oil in a Dutch oven over medium-high heat. Add the onion, celery, and carrots, and cook, stirring often, until softened, about 5 minutes. Next add the mushrooms and sauté for an additional 2 to 3 minutes.

5. Add the remaining 3 tablespoons of white flour, the remaining ½ teaspoon of rosemary, and the thyme, sage, and pepper, and cook, stirring constantly, for 1 minute. Gradually whisk in the reserved chicken stock and bring to boil. Reduce the heat to low and simmer, uncovered, stirring often, for about 5 minutes.

6. Stir in the potatoes and cooked chicken pieces, along with any accumulated juices from the plate. Drop the dumpling dough onto the stew by tablespoons, leaving space around each dumpling so they don't touch. Cover and cook without lifting the lid for 10 to 15 minutes, or until a toothpick inserted in the dumplings comes out clean. Serve immediately. Serves 4 to 6.

Baked Mumbai Chicken with Rice

gluten-free
dairy-free

This chicken baked with brown rice, almonds, coconuts, and curry spice was a family favourite while my children were still living at home, and it's still much requested when they come home for a visit.

- ½ cup slivered almonds
- ½ cup desiccated coconut
- 2 to 3 tbsp. sunflower oil
- 3 lbs. skinless chicken, cubed
- 1 large onion, diced
- 3 cloves garlic, minced
- 2 cups uncooked brown rice
- 2 tbsp. curry powder
- 1 tsp. paprika
- 1 tbsp. Bragg Liquid Aminos
- 1 cup Thompson raisins
- 4 cups chicken stock

1. Preheat the oven to 375°F.

2. Place the almonds and coconut in a small, dry skillet, and cook, stirring often, over medium heat until toasted. Remove from the heat and set aside.

3. Heat the oil in an ovenproof Dutch oven over medium-high heat. Add the chicken pieces in batches and cook, stirring often, for 4 to 5 minutes, or until browned. Transfer the cooked chicken to a plate.

4. Pour an extra tablespoon of oil to the Dutch oven if needed. Add the onion and garlic and sauté for 3 to 4 minutes. Stirring after each addition, add the uncooked brown rice, curry powder, paprika, Bragg's, raisins, chicken stock, and all but 2 tablespoons of the toasted almonds and coconut. Bring to a boil. Reduce the heat to low and simmer, covered, for 10 minutes.

5. Place the chicken pieces on top of the rice, cover, and place the Dutch oven into the preheated oven. Bake for 1 hour, or until the chicken juice runs clear and the rice is tender. Garnish with the remaining toasted almond and coconut mix before serving. Serves 4.

Normandy Chicken

gluten-free

The Normandy region of France, which is north of Paris and follows 360 miles of the English channel, is known for its cream, butter, cheeses, apples, and apple brandy. In our version of Normandy Chicken, we use less butter than the traditional method and low-fat sour cream.

- **2 tbsp. butter, divided**
- **2 cooking apples (Fuji or Jonagold), cored and sliced into wedges**
- **4 skinless chicken legs or breasts**
- **1 large onion, peeled and sliced into wedges**
- **3 stalks celery, chopped**
- **½ cup apple brandy or Calvados**
- **2 cups apple cider**
- **1 tsp. dried thyme**
- **½ cup low-fat sour cream**
- **sea salt to taste**
- **freshly ground pepper to taste**

1. Heat 1 tablespoon of the butter in a large skillet over medium heat. Add the apple slices and sauté, turning occasionally, until they turn a little brown around the edges. Set the apples aside on paper towels to drain.

2. Melt the remaining tablespoon of butter in the skillet. Add the chicken pieces and fry until golden, about 3 to 5 minutes on each side. Remove the chicken from the pan and set aside.

3. Add the onion and celery and increase the heat to medium-high. Sauté, stirring occasionally, until they are caramelized, about 5 to 8 minutes. Add the brandy to the pan. Using a wooden spoon, scrape any remaining brown bits off the bottom of the pan.

4. Return the chicken to the pan and let the sauce boil until it has reduced by about half. Add the cider and thyme and bring to a boil. Cook, uncovered, for 20 to 25 minutes, or until the liquid has again reduced by half.

5. Add the apples back into the skillet. Place the sour cream in a medium-sized mixing bowl and stir in a ladle full of the hot liquid from the skillet to it to temper it. Pour the sour cream into the pan and stir just until heated through.

6. Season with sea salt and freshly ground pepper to taste. Serves 4.

Chocolatey Chicken Mole

gluten-free
dairy-free

Mole (pronounced MOLE–lay), is a particularly delicious example of Mexican cuisine. I love the complex layering of flavours in Mexican cooking, especially in this dish, where browned chicken pieces are simmered in a spicy tomato and chocolate sauce. (And I love chocolate!)

- 1 tbsp. sunflower oil
- 3 lbs. bone-in chicken thighs or legs
- 1 bay leaf
- ¼ tsp. freshly ground pepper
- 1 tbsp. chipotle pepper, minced
- ½ tsp. paprika
- ½ tsp. ground cloves
- ½ tsp. ground cinnamon
- 1 onion, chopped
- 2 cloves garlic, minced
- 2 cups diced tomatoes
- 2 tsp. brown sugar
- 1 cup chicken stock
- ¼ cup semisweet chocolate chips
- ¼ cup raisins
- 2 tbsp. sesame seeds

1. Heat the oil in a large pot or Dutch oven over medium-high heat. Add the chicken pieces and cook until browned on all sides, about 10 minutes. Remove the chicken from the pot and set aside.

2. Reduce the heat to medium and stir in the bay leaf, pepper, chipotle pepper, paprika, cloves, and cinnamon. Cook until fragrant, about 30 seconds. Add the onion and garlic and stir until the onion has softened, about 5 minutes.

3. Stir in the tomatoes, brown sugar, and chicken stock and bring to a simmer over medium-high heat. Once the liquid is simmering, stir in the chocolate chips. Continue stirring until the chocolate chips have melted, then return the chicken pieces to the pot.

4. Reduce the heat to medium-low, cover, and let simmer until the chicken is tender and no longer pink at the bone, about 25 to 30 minutes. Stir in the raisins and cook for 3 minutes longer. Garnish with the sesame seeds before serving. Serves 4 to 6.

Stuffed Chicken Breasts: My Way or Your Way

gluten-free

Feta and spinach–stuffed chicken breasts were well-sought-after during my meal delivery days. Below is the original recipe, along with some mix-and-match ideas for any kind of stuffed chicken breast you desire (or have the ingredients for).

- 1 (10 oz.) package frozen spinach, thawed and drained well
- 1 cup. crumbled feta cheese
- 2 cloves garlic, minced
- 1 tbsp. Parmesan cheese
- sea salt to taste
- freshly ground pepper to taste
- 4 boneless, skinless chicken breasts, halved widthwise
- 1 to 2 tbsp. olive oil

1. Preheat the oven to 375°F.

2. In a medium-sized mixing bowl, combine the spinach with the feta cheese, garlic, Parmesan cheese, salt, and pepper.*

3. Using a sharp knife, cut a horizontal slit through thickest portion of each chicken breast half to form a pocket. Fill each chicken pocket with some of the feta stuffing mix. Place the stuffed chicken breasts on a lightly greased baking dish with the stuffed ends pressed together to keep the filling in. Brush the outside of the chicken breasts with the olive oil.

4. Place the baking dish on the top shelf of the preheated oven and bake for 40 to 45 minutes, or until the chicken is firm and the juices run clear.

*If you take half of this stuffing and put it into another bowl and set it aside, it won't get contaminated. This way, if you have extra, it can be saved or frozen.

Here are some other stuffing suggestions for you to mix and match. Go crazy!

- **RICOTTA CHEESE**
- **GOAT CHEESE**
- **BLUE CHEESE**
- **BRIE OR CAMEMBERT CHEESE**
- **ASIAGO CHEESE**
- **SWISS CHEESE**
- **SUN-DRIED TOMATOES**
- **SAUTÉED MUSHROOMS**

- **ROASTED BELL PEPPERS**
- **FRESH OR DRIED HERBS**
- **BACON BITS**
- **FIGS**
- **DRIED CRANBERRIES**
- **TOASTED NUTS**
- **PESTO**

Chicken à la Karin

There's no need to feel guilty over this classic creamy combination of chicken, peppers, and mushrooms. Our healthier version is fit for any king or queen. Serve over rice, whole wheat egg noodles, or Karin's Coveted Biscuits (page 182).

- **2 tbsp. sunflower oil, divided**
- **3 to 4 boneless, skinless chicken breasts, cut into 1-inch cubes**
- **12 to 14 button mushrooms, sliced**
- **1 green bell pepper, sliced**
- **1 red bell pepper, sliced**
- **½ tsp. sea salt**
- **½ tsp. freshly ground pepper**
- **1 cup white wine**
- **½ cup unbleached white flour**
- **1 cup chicken stock**
- **1 cup skim milk**
- **2 to 3 green onions, sliced**

1. Heat 1 tablespoon of the oil in a large skillet over medium-high heat. Add the chicken in batches and cook, stirring occasionally, until lightly browned, about 2 to 4 minutes. Transfer the cooked chicken to a plate.

2. Heat the remaining tablespoon of oil in the skillet. Add the mushrooms, green and red peppers, sea salt, and pepper and cook, stirring often, until the vegetables have softened, about 3 to 5 minutes.

3. Pour in the white wine and bring to a boil, stirring constantly to scrape up any browned bits from the bottom of the skillet.

4. In a medium-sized bowl, make a slurry by whisking the flour with the chicken stock until smooth. Add the slurry to the skillet and stir until well blended. Add the milk and bring to a boil. Reduce the heat to low and simmer, stirring often, until the mixture is the consistency of cream.

5. Return the chicken to the skillet and keep simmering, stirring often, for 10 to 15 minutes, or until the chicken is firm and the juices run clear. Stir in the green onions and serve immediately. Serves 4 to 6.

Chicken and Vegetable Shepherd's Pie

When I think of this meal, I think of Dodie, who is a client-turned-friend. When this extremely busy lady needs some good comfort food, this dish is her answer. Here's to you, Dod! xoxo

- **5 cups chicken stock**
- **2 to 3 lbs. skinned chicken thighs and drumsticks**
- **9 to 12 potatoes, peeled and cut into 2-inch cubes**
- **1 tbsp. sunflower oil**
- **1 large onion, sliced**
- **1½ cups sliced celery**
- **3 small carrots, peeled and sliced**
- **1 cup mushrooms, halved**

- **3 tbsp. unbleached white flour**
- **½ tsp. dried thyme**
- **½ tsp. dried sage**
- **½ tsp. dried rosemary**
- **¼ tsp. sea salt**
- **¼ tsp. freshly ground pepper**
- **2 tbsp. chopped fresh parsley**

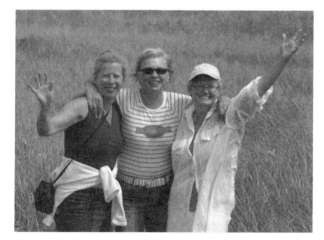

Me with my friends Gale and Dodie, having a blast in the Magdalen Islands.

1. In a large pot, bring chicken stock to boil over medium-high heat. Reduce the heat to medium-low. Add the chicken, cover, and simmer until the juices run clear when the chicken is pierced, about 30 minutes.

2. While the chicken is cooking, place the potatoes in a separate large pot and cover with water. Bring to a boil over high heat. Reduce the heat to low and simmer for 20 to 25 minutes, or until the potatoes are easily pierced with a fork. Drain, reserving 1 cup of the cooking liquid. Return the potatoes to the pot and mash until very soft. Add the reserved potato liquid if needed. Season with sea salt and pepper to taste. Set aside.

3. Preheat the oven to 375°F.

4. When the chicken is cooked, transfer it to a plate using a slotted spoon, reserving the chicken stock. Let the chicken cool, and then remove the meat from bones. Cut the meat into bite-sized chunks.

5. Heat the oil in a Dutch oven over medium-high heat. Add the onion, celery, and carrots and cook, stirring often, until softened, about 5 minutes. Next add the mushrooms and sauté for an additional 2 to 3 minutes.

6. Add the flour, thyme, sage, rosemary, salt, and pepper and cook, stirring constantly, for 1 minute. Gradually whisk in the reserved chicken stock. Bring to boil and continue to stir until the sauce has thickened, about 2 to 3 minutes. Reduce the heat to medium-low, and let simmer, uncovered, stirring often, for about 5 minutes, or until it has reduced to the consistency of thick cream. Return the chicken and any accumulated juices from the plate to the pot.

7. Spoon the chicken mixture into a lightly greased 9" × 13" baking pan. Dollop spoonfuls of the mashed potato on top. Sprinkle the fresh parsley over the potatoes.

8. Bake in the preheated oven for 35 to 45 minutes, or until the potatoes are lightly browned. If the potatoes haven't browned after 45 minutes, place them under the broiler for 2 minutes or until golden brown. Serve immediately. Serves 6 to 8.

Peruvian Roasted Chicken "El Pollo Rico"

gluten-free
dairy-free

"El pollo rico" means "delicious chicken," and this recipe certainly is that. This chicken dish became hugely popular along the East Coast of the United States a few years ago. It is a tasty way to cook chicken with enough flavour to satisfy anyone, but still mild enough to satisfy everyone.

- **4 tbsp. white vinegar**
- **3 tbsp. white wine**
- **3 tbsp. sunflower oil**
- **3 cloves garlic, minced**
- **1½ tbsp. ground cumin**
- **2 tbsp. paprika**
- **2 tsp. freshly ground pepper**
- **1 tsp. sea salt**
- **1 lemon, zest and juice**
- **4 cups cold water**
- **1 (4 lb.) whole chicken, trimmed of excess fat**
- **½ cup mayonnaise**
- **2 tbsp. mustard**
- **2 tbsp. lime juice**

1. In a medium-sized mixing bowl, combine the vinegar, white wine, oil, garlic, cumin, paprika, pepper, and salt. Mix well to form a paste. Set aside.

2. In a separate large mixing bowl, combine the lemon zest and juice with the cold water. Wash the chicken thoroughly in the lemon water.

3. Place the chicken in a large zippered freezer bag. Pour the spice paste over the chicken. Coat the chicken completely with the spice mixture, rubbing into every surface. Try to get the paste under the skin as much as possible.

4. Seal the bag and place the chicken in the refrigerator for at least 2 hours or more. The longer it marinates the more flavour it gets.

5. While the chicken is marinating, combine the mayonnaise, mustard, and lime juice in a small bowl. Cover and store in the fridge until ready to serve.

6. When the chicken has finished marinating, preheat the oven to 350°F.

7. Place the marinated chicken in a lightly greased roasting pan. Place the pan in the preheated oven and roast for approximately 1½ hours, basting occasionally. Test the chicken for doneness with a meat thermometer in the thickest part of the thigh. The chicken is done when it reaches 165°F. Let the chicken stand for 5 to 7 minutes before carving.

8. Carve the chicken and serve with rice, the mayonnaise and mustard dipping sauce, and Aji Verde (page 72). Serves 4 to 6.

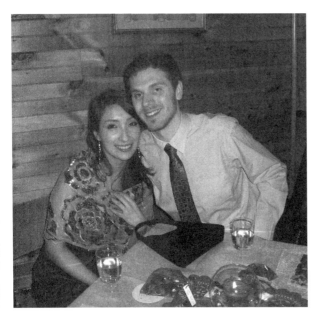

This is my son Elliot and, at this writing, my daughter-in-law-to-be, Yanet. Yanet is from Peru. The two are planning to get married in the summer of 2013. We are so happy!

Awesome Oven-Barbecued Chicken

gluten-free
dairy-free

We served this quite often in the Eat Well kitchen, but I forgot all about it until Lori McDonald, who toiled many hard hours in the kitchen, reminded me. The base is our Eat Well Tomato Sauce (page 67). Make a batch of it ahead of time and freeze what you don't need.

- **3 lbs. chicken pieces (breasts, thighs, or legs)**
- **2 cups Eat Well Tomato Sauce (page 67)**
- **2 tbsp. brown sugar**
- **1 tsp. ground cumin**
- **1 tsp. chopped chipotle pepper or chipotle powder**
- **2 to 3 drops liquid smoke**

1. Preheat the oven to 350°F.

2. Place the chicken pieces in a lightly greased 9" × 13" baking pan.

3. In a medium-sized mixing bowl, combine the tomato sauce with the brown sugar, cumin, chipotle, and liquid smoke. Pour the sauce over the chicken.

4. Bake, basting and stirring occasionally, for 45 to 55 minutes, or until the chicken is firm and starting to fall off the bone.

5. Serve with Oven Potato or Sweet Potato Fries (page 63). Serves 6.

Mango Coconut Curried Chicken

gluten-free
dairy-free

Lori McDonald, who I was lucky enough to work with in the Eat Well kitchen for several years, loves this easy-to-make meal. The exotic flavours of the mango, coconut, and curry make this chicken dish taste like the tropics.

- **1 to 2 tbsp. sunflower oil**
- **4 boneless, skinless chicken breasts**
- **1 mango, peeled and cubed, or 1 cup frozen mango**
- **1 cup coconut milk**
- **1 tsp. lime juice**
- **2 tsp. curry powder**
- **½ tsp. sea salt**
- **½ tsp. freshly ground pepper**
- **1 tbsp. chopped fresh cilantro or parsley**

1. Heat 1 tablespoon of the oil in a large skillet over medium-high heat. Add the chicken breasts and cook 4 to 5 minutes, or until browned on both sides, adding the remaining tablespoon of oil if needed. Transfer the cooked chicken to a plate.

2. Add the mango, coconut milk, lime juice, curry powder, sea salt, and pepper to the skillet and stir to combine. Return the chicken and cook over medium-high heat, covered, for 40 to 50 minutes, or until the juices run clear. Garnish with the cilantro or parsley before serving. Serves 4.

Ann's Maple Chicken

gluten-free

While I had my catering service, one of my clients, Ann, shared this recipe with me. We tried it, and it was a hit—it was requested on a regular basis. The original recipe suggests serving it with pasta, but you can substitute rice for a gluten-free option.

- **1 tbsp. sunflower oil**
- **4 boneless, skinless chicken breasts, sliced into 2-inch cubes**
- **1 red bell pepper, chopped**
- **1 yellow pepper, chopped**
- **1 green bell pepper, chopped**
- **1 cup sliced button mushrooms**
- **¼ cup pure maple syrup**
- **2½ tbsp. tandoori curry paste**
- **1 cup whipping cream**

1. Heat the oil in a large skillet over medium heat. Add the chicken in batches if needed, and cook for 2 to 3 minutes on each side, or until browned on all sides. Transfer the chicken to a plate.

2. Add the red, yellow, and green peppers and the mushrooms to the skillet and cook for 4 to 5 minutes, or until soft. Return the chicken to the skillet and cook for 3 minutes. Stir in the maple syrup and cook for 5 more minutes.

3. Stir in the tandoori curry paste and the whipping cream. Reduce the heat to low and simmer, uncovered, for 10 to 15 minutes, or until the sauce reaches the thickness of cream.

4. Serve over rice or penne pasta. Serves 4 to 6.

Here's the Beef!

We were all about including "every body" in the Eat Well kitchen, so there were always a couple of beef choices on our weekly catering menu. Your kids will love the Scoobi Doo Pasta with Meat Sauce and Cheese *(page 170)* or Savoury Meat and Vegetable Swirl *(page 171)*. And if you are entertaining and want to impress, you can't go wrong with Morgan's Stuffed Steak *(page 177)*.

Greek-Style Shepherd's Pie

gluten-free

This is a bit of a twist on the traditional Shepherd's pie that Mom used to make.

- **5 large unpeeled potatoes, washed and quartered**
- **½ cup skim milk**
- **2 tbsp. olive oil**
- **1 tsp. sea salt**
- **1 tsp. dried oregano, divided**
- **1½ lb. extra-lean ground beef or ground turkey**
- **1 onion, chopped**
- **2 cloves garlic, minced**
- **½ tsp. freshly ground pepper**
- **½ lemon, zest and juice**
- **2 large tomatoes, sliced**
- **½ cup shredded mozzarella cheese**
- **½ cup crumbled feta cheese**
- **1 (300 g) package frozen spinach, thawed and drained**

1. Place the potatoes in a large pot and cover with water. Cook over medium-high heat for 20 to 25 minutes, or until tender. Drain well, reserving the cooking liquid. Return the potatoes to the pot and add the milk, olive oil, sea salt, and ½ teaspoon of the oregano. Mash well. Stir in some of the reserved cooking liquid to make the consistency soft and smooth, if needed. Set aside.

2. Preheat the oven to 350°F.

3. Place the beef or turkey, onion, garlic, pepper, and the remaining ½ teaspoon of oregano in a large skillet over medium-high heat. Cook, stirring occasionally, for 4 to 5 minutes, or until the meat is browned. Stir in the lemon juice and zest.

4. Place the meat mixture in the bottom of a lightly greased 9" × 13" baking pan. Layer the tomato slices over the beef. Sprinkle the mozzarella and feta cheeses evenly over the tomatoes. Spread the spinach evenly over the cheese layer. Spoon the mashed potatoes on top and smooth them out.

5. Bake in the preheated oven for 45 minutes, or until the potatoes begin to brown. Allow to cool for 5 minutes before serving. Serves 6 to 8.

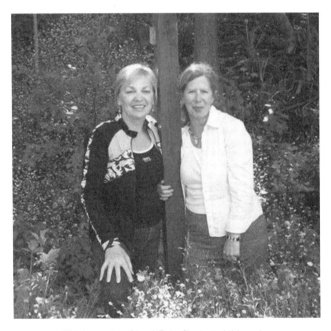

This is my dear friend Gale. She tested this recipe and suggested substituting the ground beef or turkey for ground lamb. Thank you, Gale!

Southwest Beef and Vegetable-Stuffed Peppers

vegetarian option

What better way to use those large, sweet bell peppers during the harvest season than with this easy and delicious spicy beef–stuffed pepper recipe? The sweetness of the peppers plays off the spicy ground beef used to stuff them, and the result is a colourful combination perfect for a festive meal.

Replace the ground beef with veggie ground round for a vegetarian version.

- **6 whole bell peppers (your choice of colours)**
- **1 lb. extra-lean ground beef**
- **½ cup chopped onion**
- **½ cup chopped celery**
- **2 cloves garlic, minced**
- **3 cups homemade salsa (page 68) or store-bought salsa, divided**
- **1 cup corn kernels**
- **1 cup cooked brown rice**
- **1 tsp. ground cumin**
- **1 tsp. dried oregano**
- **1 tsp. chili powder**
- **sea salt to taste**
- **freshly ground pepper to taste**
- **1½ cups shredded Mexican cheese blend***

1. Preheat the oven to 350°F.

2. Rinse the peppers under cold water. Remove the tops, seeds, and membranes. Chop the edible part of the tops.

3. Place the beef, onion, celery, garlic, and chopped pepper tops in a large skillet over medium-high heat. Cook, stirring often, for 6 to 10 minutes, or until the beef is evenly browned and the vegetables are soft. Stir in the corn, rice, cumin, oregano, chili powder, salt, pepper, and 2 cups of the salsa.

4. Spoon equal amounts of the filling into the cored peppers. Arrange them standing upright in a lightly greased baking dish. Pour the remaining cup of salsa on top.

5. Bake in the preheated oven, occasionally basting the peppers with the salsa, for 50 minutes. If you would like to add cheese, remove the peppers from the oven and sprinkle them with the grated cheese blend. Return to the oven and bake for 10 more minutes. Serves 6.

*Optional

Baked Lebanese-Spiced Kibbee

gluten-free option
dairy-free

In this classic Middle Eastern recipe, ground beef is layered with pine nuts and baked. If you wish to make it gluten-free, replace the bulgur and hot water with 1 cup of cooked quinoa. This is tasty served with Mjadra (page 116) and/or Haida's Tabouli Salad (page 49).

- **½ cup bulgur**
- **½ cup hot water**
- **½ tsp. dried mint**
- **¼ tsp. ground allspice**
- **¼ tsp. ground pepper**
- **¼ tsp. ground cinnamon**
- **¼ tsp. sea salt**
- **1 onion, finely chopped**
- **2 tbsp. chopped fresh parsley**
- **1 lb. lean ground beef**
- **3 tbsp. pine nuts or slivered almonds, toasted**

1. Place the bulgur in a small mixing bowl and cover with the hot water. Soak until the bulgur expands and cools, about 10 minutes.

2. Place the bulgur, mint, allspice, pepper, cinnamon, salt, onion, parsley, and beef in the bowl of a food processor. Process until well mixed, about 1 minute.

3. Divide the mixture in two and press one half into the bottom of a lightly greased baking dish. Sprinkle 2 tablespoons of the toasted pine nuts over the meat. Layer the remaining beef on top, patting it down firmly. Cut the kibbee into 3-inch squares and then cut each of the squares in half diagonally. Garnish with the remaining pine nuts.

4. Bake in the preheated oven for 30 to 35 minutes, or until the beef is fully browned Serves 4.

Perfect Pizza Rustica

We amazed many of our customers with this delicious and appealing fare. We served it hot at the farmers' market and it always sold out. Another time it was a great hit at my friend Gale's 50th birthday party, although Gale was the greatest hit of all.

- **3½ cups unbleached white flour**
- **¾ lb. cold butter, cut into pieces**
- **¼ cup cold shortening, cut into pieces**
- **1 tsp. salt**
- **4 large whole eggs, divided, plus 4 eggs, yolks only**
- **2 to 4 tbsp. ice water**
- **1 tbsp. sunflower oil**
- **1 lb. ground beef, turkey, or sausage (casings removed)**

- **1 tsp. minced garlic**
- **1 cup Eat Well Tomato Sauce (page 67)**
- **1 (10-ounce) package frozen cut-leaf spinach, thawed and drained**
- **1 (15-ounce) container whole milk ricotta**
- **2 cups shredded mozzarella cheese**
- **⅓ cup plus 2 tbsp. freshly grated Parmesan cheese, divided**

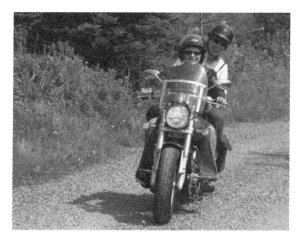

My friend Gale and I took a girl trip on her motorbike to the Magdalen Islands. Oh, what fun!

1. Process the flour, butter, shortening, and salt in a food processor until the mixture resembles a coarse meal. Beat 3 of the whole eggs in a separate small bowl and add to the mixture in the food processor. Process to blend. With the machine running, add the ice water 1 tablespoon at a time until a dough forms.

2. Gather the dough into a ball. Divide the dough into 2 pieces, with the first piece twice as large as the second piece. Flatten the dough pieces into disks. Wrap the dough disks in plastic wrap and refrigerate until the dough is firm enough to roll out, about 30 minutes.

3. Preheat the oven to 375°F.

4. Heat the oil in a large, heavy frying pan over medium heat. Add the ground meat and garlic and sauté for 5 minutes, or until the meat is golden brown. Stir in the tomato sauce and spinach. Set aside to cool.

5. Place the 4 egg yolks in a large mixing bowl and beat lightly. Stir in the ricotta, mozzarella, and ⅓ cup of the Parmesan cheese. Add the cooled meat and spinach sauce and stir to combine. Set aside.

6. Remove the pastry dough from the refrigerator. Roll out the larger piece of dough on a lightly floured work surface to a 17-inch round. Press the dough into the bottom of a 9-inch springform pan. Trim the dough overhang to 1 inch. Spoon the ricotta, meat, and sauce mixture into the dough-lined pan.

7. Roll out the remaining piece of dough into a 12-inch round. Lay the dough over the filling. Pinch the edges of the two rounds of dough together to seal, and then crimp the dough edges decoratively.

8. Beat the remaining whole egg in a small bowl and brush evenly over the pastry top. Sprinkle the remaining 2 tablespoons of Parmesan over the pastry.

9. Bake on the bottom rack of the preheated oven until the crust is golden brown, about 1 hour. Let stand for 15 minutes. Release the springform ring and transfer the pizza to a platter. Cut into wedges to serve. Serves 6 to 8.

Scoobi Doo Pasta with Meat Sauce and Cheese

I could not sell enough of this meal—it was by far the most popular with our meat-eating customers.

Scoobi doo is pasta formed in a spiral tube shape. It is also known as cavatappi or tortiglione.

- 1 ½ lbs. lean ground beef
- ½ tsp. sea salt
- ½ tsp. freshly ground pepper
- 4 cups scoobi doo pasta
- 4 cups Eat Well Tomato Sauce (page 67)
- 1 cup shredded mozzarella cheese
- 1 cup shredded cheddar cheese
- 1 tbsp. dried parsley

1. Preheat the oven to 350°F.

2. Crumble the ground beef into a large skillet over medium-high heat. Season with the salt and pepper. Cook, stirring frequently, for 5 to 6 minutes, or until browned.

3. While the beef is cooking, bring a large pot of water to a boil. Add the pasta and cook until tender, about 8 minutes. Drain, but don't rinse.

4. Return the pasta to the pot. Add the ground beef and the tomato sauce and stir until combined. Pour the pasta into a lightly greased 9" × 11" baking pan. Top with the mozzarella cheese. Spread the cheddar cheese in a layer on top of the mozzarella. Sprinkle with the dried parsley.

5. Bake, uncovered, in the preheated oven for 30 minutes, or until bubbly and heated through. Serves 6 to 8.

My buds Callum and Tristan loved the scoobi doo pasta so much, they came to the kitchen to make it.

Savoury Meat and Vegetable Swirl

vegetarian option

This savoury pastry is a great thing to make when you want to clean out your fridge. You can use ground beef, sausage, ground turkey, or chicken and whichever vegetables you have that are looking for attention. It is also a great time to use up your leftover cheese chunks. For a vegetarian option, replace the meat with veggie ground round, mashed beans, or more vegetables.

- 1 lb. ground beef, turkey, or sausage (casings removed)
- 1 onion, diced
- 2 cloves garlic, minced
- 2 cups diced assorted vegetables (carrots, peppers, broccoli, mushrooms, etc.)
- 1 tsp. dried oregano
- 1 tsp. dried basil
- 1 tsp. dried thyme
- 1 tsp. Bragg Liquid Aminos
- ½ tsp. freshly ground pepper
- 2 cups Eat Well Tomato Sauce (page 67) or your favourite tomato sauce
- 1 cup unbleached white flour
- 1 cup whole wheat flour
- 4 tsp. baking powder
- ½ tsp. sea salt
- ½ tsp. Italian seasoning
- ¼ cup cold butter or shortening
- 1 egg, beaten
- ¾ cup milk
- 2 cups grated cheese (your choice)

1. Place the meat, onion, and garlic in a large skillet over medium heat and cook, stirring occasionally, for 5 to 7 minutes, or until the meat is browned. Add the assorted vegetables, oregano, basil, thyme, Bragg's, and pepper and stir to combine. Add the tomato sauce and bring to a boil. Reduce the heat to low and simmer, uncovered, for 10 to 15 minutes, or until the mixture is thick like stew. Remove from heat and let cool.

2. Preheat the oven to 425°F.

3. In a large mixing bowl, sift together the white and whole wheat flower, baking powder, sea salt, and Italian seasoning. Cut in the butter and combine. Add the egg and milk and mix well. Bring the dough together in ball. Place the dough ball on a lightly floured work surface and roll out into a 9" × 12" rectangle.*

4. Spread the meat filling onto the dough rectangle to ½ inch from the edges. Sprinkle half of the cheese evenly over the top. Wet the edges of the pastry and carefully roll up like a jelly roll.

5. Place the cut side of the roll down on a lightly greased or parchment-lined baking sheet. Sprinkle with the remaining cheese. Bake in the preheated oven for 30 minutes, or until the crust is golden brown. Slice into 2-inch pieces. Let stand for 5 minutes before serving. Serves 4 to 6.

*Note: Rolling the pastry out onto parchment paper or splitting the dough in two pieces may make it easier when you have to transfer the roll to the baking sheet later on.

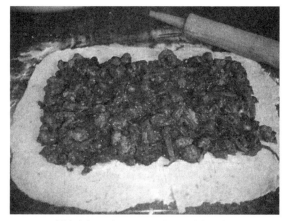

This is how the meat and vegetable swirl should look before you roll it up.

Hachée (Dutch Beef and Onion Stew)

dairy-free

This meal is part of my heritage. My mom made it for us on a regular basis. I've integrated it into our Eat Well menu and we've developed quite a few Dutch food fans.

- **2 large onions, thinly sliced**
- **¼ cup butter**
- **¼ cup unbleached white flour**
- **2 cups beef stock**
- **3 bay leaves**
- **5 cloves**
- **1 tbsp. vinegar**
- **½ lb. sliced leftover cooked beef**
- **2 tbsp. cornstarch**
- **2 tbsp. water**
- **freshly ground pepper to taste**
- **Worcestershire sauce to taste**

1. Melt the butter in a large skillet over medium heat. Add the onions and sauté, stirring often, for 4 to 5 minutes, or until caramelized and browned. Add the flour and stir until smooth. Gradually pour in the cold stock, stirring constantly until thickened to the consistency of gravy. Stir in the bay leaves and cloves. Reduce the heat to low and simmer, covered, for 5 minutes.

2. Stir in the vinegar and the diced meat. Simmer, covered, for 1 hour to cook off the flour taste.

3. In a small bowl, mix the cornstarch and water to make a slurry. Stir the slurry into the stew. Simmer, stirring constantly, for 5 minutes, or until thickened.

4. Season to taste with pepper and Worcestershire sauce. Serve with boiled potatoes. Serves 4.

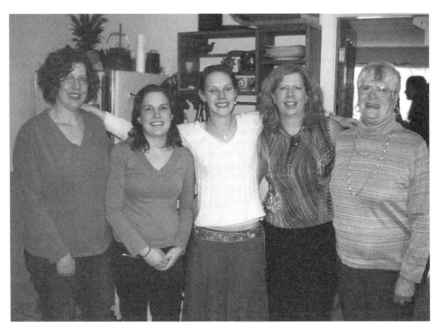

That is my sweet mom on the far right. She is with her two daughters and two granddaughters. Mom was a terrific cook—her favourite ingredient was love!

Spicy Szechwan Beef

gluten-free
dairy-free

The complex, spicy meal goes well with Asian-style noodles or brown rice.

- ½ tsp. Szechwan peppercorns (available at any Asian grocery)
- 1 (2-inch) piece cinnamon stick, broken up
- ½ tsp. aniseed
- 1 to 2 tbsp. sunflower oil
- 1½ lbs. tender beef steak, sliced into strips
- 2 garlic cloves, crushed
- 2 tsp. grated fresh unpeeled ginger
- ½ tsp. cayenne pepper
- 4 green onions, sliced thin
- 2 cups thinly sliced bok choy
- 1 tbsp. Bragg Liquid Aminos
- 1 tbsp. rice wine vinegar

1. Place the peppercorns, cinnamon pieces, and aniseed in a large, dry skillet over medium-high heat. Toast, shaking the pan constantly, until they begin to smoke. Let cool and grind in a spice grinder. Set aside.

2. Heat the oil in the skillet over high heat. Add half the beef and cook, stirring constantly, for 2 to 3 minutes, or until browned. Transfer to a bowl. Repeat with the remaining beef.

3. Return the cooked beef from the bowl to the skillet. Stir in the garlic, ginger, cayenne, and green onions and stir-fry for 1 to 2 minutes, or until the beef and spices are well combined. Stir in the bok choy, Bragg's, and rice wine vinegar. Reduce the heat to medium and cook for 2 to 3 minutes, or until the bok choy has wilted. Serves 4.

Beef Satay

gluten-free
dairy-free

This is another Indonesian specialty of my mom's that was a real treat while growing up. It was my dad's favourite. You can exchange the beef with chicken or tofu. Serve this with our Spicy Thai Peanut Sauce (page 71) and Indonesian Nasi Goreng with Tofu (page 80).

- ½ medium onion, chopped
- 3 cloves garlic, peeled
- 1 tbsp. minced fresh unpeeled ginger
- 1 tbsp. chopped fresh lemongrass
- 1 tbsp. brown sugar
- 2 tsp. sambal oelek*
- 1 tsp. ground coriander
- ½ cup Bragg Liquid Aminos
- 2 tbsp. sesame oil
- 1 tbsp. fresh lemon juice
- 1½ lbs. beef sirloin, trimmed of fat and sliced into strips
- 8 to 10 metal or bamboo** skewers

1. Place the onion, garlic, ginger, lemongrass, brown sugar, sambal oelek, coriander, Bragg's, sesame oil, and lemon juice in the bowl of a food processor and pulse until smooth.

2. Place the beef slices in a nonreactive container and pour the marinade over the beef. Stir until all slices are covered. Refrigerate 1 to 2 hours or overnight.

3. Preheat the grill or barbecue to medium-high.

4. Thread the marinated beef strips onto the skewers by fanning them back and forth loosely, retaining the marinating liquid.

5. Lay the skewered beef on the preheated grill. Cook, basting often with the marinade, for 2 to 4 minutes on each side, or until the meat is browned and feels firm. Serves 4.

*Sambal oelek is a red chili paste available at most Asian markets.

**If using bamboo skewers, soak them in water for at least 30 minutes before using them.

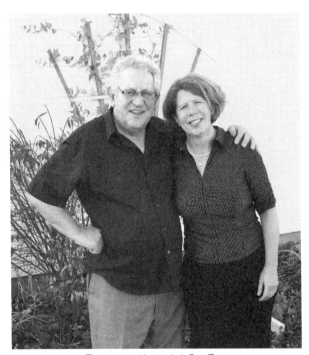

This is me with my dad, Con Zaat.

Teriyaki Beef and Vegetables

gluten-free
dairy-free

If preferred, you can swap the beef in this recipe for equal amounts of chicken or tofu. Serve this dish with noodles or brown rice.

- **2 tbsp. brown sugar**
- **1 tbsp. cornstarch**
- **2 tbsp. Bragg Liquid Aminos**
- **1 tbsp. rice vinegar**
- **3 tbsp. water**
- **1 to 2 tbsp. vegetable oil**
- **1 lb. beef stir-fry strips**
- **1 onion, sliced**
- **3 garlic cloves, minced**
- **1 tbsp. minced fresh unpeeled ginger**
- **1 cup dried shiitake mushrooms, rehydrated with 1 cup water (reserve liquid)**
- **4 cups mixed sliced vegetables (broccoli, coloured bell peppers, carrots, baby bok choy, etc.)**
- **1 tbsp. sesame oil**
- **1 tbsp. toasted sesame seeds (a mix of black and white if you have them)**

1. In a medium-sized mixing bowl, stir together the brown sugar, cornstarch, Bragg's, rice vinegar, and water. Set aside.

2. Heat 1 tablespoon of the oil in a large wok or skillet over high heat. Add half the beef and stir-fry until browned, about 4 minutes per batch. Transfer the cooked beef to a bowl. Add another tablespoon of oil if needed and repeat the stir-frying steps with the remaining beef. Set the cooked beef aside.

3. Reduce the heat to medium. Add the onion, garlic, and ginger to the wok and stir-fry until fragrant, about 1 to 2 minutes. Drain the mushrooms, reserving the liquid, and add them to the wok along with the remaining vegetables. Stir-fry for 3 to 5 minutes, or until the vegetables are slightly tender but still crisp.

4. Stir in the reserved mushroom liquid. Re-stir the cornstarch mixture and slowly add it to the wok. Stir the mixture constantly until the sauce is glossy and thickened, about 4 minutes. Stir in the sesame oil.

5. Garnish with the sesame seeds before serving. Serves 4.

Creamy Beef with Chanterelles and Rosemary

gluten-free

We are lucky to live in PEI, where we can go into the woods and find lovely chanterelle mushrooms. Usually you can detect their aroma before you see them. In this dish, the earthy chanterelles and fragrant rosemary come together in some wonderful flavours.

- **2 tbsp. olive oil, divided**
- **1½ lbs. sirloin steak, trimmed of fat and sliced into thin strips**
- **3 tbsp. brandy**
- **2 shallots, finely chopped**
- **15-20 chanterelle mushrooms, trimmed and chopped**
- **2 tbsp. chopped fresh rosemary**
- **1 cup beef stock**
- **½ cup cream cheese**
- **1 tbsp. Dijon or other grainy mustard**
- **sea salt to taste**
- **freshly ground pepper to taste**

1. Heat 1 tablespoon of the oil in a large skillet over medium-high heat. Add the beef strips and sauté for 2 minutes, or until browned. Transfer the meat to a plate.

2. Remove the skillet from the heat and add the brandy. Stir the brandy around to loosen any brown bits in the bottom of the pan. Pour the liquid over the meat. Cover the meat with foil to keep it warm.

3. Wipe the skillet clean and heat remaining tablespoon of oil over medium-high heat. Add the shallots and sauté until slightly brown. Add the mushrooms and stir-fry gently for 3 to 4 minutes, or until softened. Stir in the rosemary and stock and simmer for 4 to 5 minutes so the liquid can take on the juices from the chanterelles.

4. Add the cream cheese, mustard, steak, and any of the brandy sauce accumulated on the bottom of the steak plate. Simmer, stirring constantly, for 2 to 3 minutes, or until the cheese has melted. Season to taste with salt and pepper.

5. Serve with potatoes or buttered noodles. Serves 4.

Morgan's Stuffed Steak

My buddy Morgan made this for his wife's birthday while we were visiting. It was delicious, so I grabbed the recipe and it soon became a favourite with my customers.

- **2 lbs. flank steak**
- **½ cup vegetable oil**
- **4 cloves garlic, minced, divided**
- **2 tbsp. vinegar**
- **2 tbsp. lemon juice**
- **¾ tsp. freshly ground pepper**
- **1 tsp. sea salt**
- **½ cup plus 1 tsp. dried oregano, divided**
- **2 cups fresh bread crumbs**
- **½ cup grated Parmesan cheese**
- **1 tsp. dried basil**
- **2 tbsp. chopped fresh parsley**
- **1 egg, beaten**

1. Score the meat by making shallow diagonal cuts at 1-inch intervals in a diamond pattern on both sides. Place the meat on a chopping block between 2 pieces of plastic wrap. Working from centre to edges, pound the steak into a rectangle shape with the flat side of a meat mallet. Remove the plastic wrap and place the steak in a shallow pan.

2. Combine the vegetable oil, 3 cloves of the garlic, the vinegar, the lemon juice, ½ teaspoon of the freshly ground pepper, ½ teaspoon of the salt, and 1 teaspoon of the dried oregano in a small mixing bowl. Pour over the steak. Marinate in the fridge from 2 hours to overnight.

3. Preheat the grill or barbecue to medium-high or turn on the broiler of the oven.

4. Combine the bread crumbs, Parmesan, basil, parsley, and egg with the remaining clove of garlic, ½ cup of dried oregano, ½ teaspoon sea salt, and ¼ teaspoon pepper in a large mixing bowl.

5. Remove the meat from the marinade, reserving the sauce for basting, and place it on a clean, dry work surface. Spread the bread crumb stuffing evenly over the centre of the steak surface, leaving a 1-inch margin on all four sides.

6. Roll the steak up from the short side. Secure the roll with wooden toothpicks or metal skewers at 1½-inch intervals. Brush the roll liberally with the reserved marinade.

7. If cooking on a grill or barbecue, place the roll directly on the grill. If cooking in the oven, place the meat on a broiler pan 3 to 4 inches from the top element. Cook to desired doneness*, turning once.

8. Remove the skewers or toothpicks, slice, and serve. Serves 4.

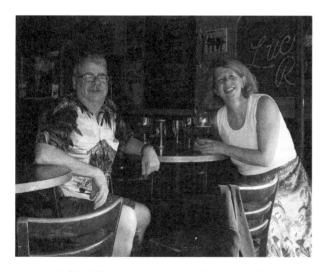

My friend Morgan and me reliving the good old days at the Lafayette in Ottawa.

*Allow 10 to 12 minutes for medium-rare, and 12 to 16 minutes for medium.

Mad for Beef Madras

gluten-free
dairy-free

This is a very authentic curry that's perfect for the Indian-food lover. Rich and pungent, it will get your taste buds hankering for more!

- **2 tbsp. ground coriander**
- **1 tbsp. ground cumin**
- **1 tsp. ground turmeric**
- **1 tsp. garam masala (page 18)**
- **½ tsp. freshly ground pepper**
- **1 tsp. chili powder**
- **2 garlic cloves, minced**
- **2 tsp. grated fresh unpeeled ginger**
- **2½ tbsp. lemon juice**
- **3 tbsp. olive oil, divided**
- **2 lbs. chuck steak, sliced into 2-inch cubes**
- **2 onions, roughly chopped**
- **2 tbsp. tomato paste**
- **1 tbsp. Bragg Liquid Aminos**
- **1 cup beef stock**
- **fresh mint leaves for garnish**

1. Combine the coriander, cumin, turmeric, garam masala, pepper, chili powder, garlic, ginger, and lemon juice in a small mixing bowl to form a paste. Set aside.

2. Heat 1 tablespoon of the oil in a large skillet over high heat. Add half the steak cubes. Cook, stirring often, for 2 to 3 minutes, or until browned. Transfer to a bowl. Repeat with remaining uncooked beef cubes.

3. Reduce the heat to medium-high and heat the remaining 2 tablespoons of oil. Add the onions and stir-fry for 2 to 3 minutes, or until soft and translucent. Add the spice paste and cook, stirring constantly, for 1 minute.

4. Return the cooked beef to the skillet and cook, stirring constantly, for 1 minute, or until the meat is coated with the spice paste. Add the tomato paste, Bragg's, and stock and bring to a boil.

5. Reduce the heat to low, cover, and simmer for 1 hour and 15 minutes, or until the beef is tender. Remove the lid and cook, uncovered, for a further 15 minutes, or until the sauce has reduced and thickened slightly.

6. Garnish with the mint leaves and serve with rice and Raita (page 76). Serves 4.

Our Better-than-Best Beef Stroganoff

gluten-free
vegetarian option

Beef Stroganoff is a great classic dish that is very easy and quick to prepare. If desired, you can substitute leftover roast beef, cut into strips, for the sirloin—just add it after the vegetables are cooked. You can also substitute the beef for chicken and the beef stock for chicken stock. Or, for a vegetarian option, use tofu and vegetable stock, and replace the Worcestershire sauce* with Bragg Liquid Aminos.

- 1½ to 2 lbs. lean sirloin beef steak, sliced into strips 2 inches long by ½ inch thick
- 2 tbsp. sunflower oil
- 3 medium onions, chopped
- 2 cloves garlic, minced
- 6 to 8 white button mushrooms, sliced
- 4 unpeeled carrots, scrubbed and sliced on the bias
- 1½ cups beef stock
- 1 tsp. Worcestershire sauce
- 2 tbsp. chopped fresh dill or 2 tsp. dried dill
- 1 cup low-fat sour cream or cream cheese**
- 2 tbsp. cornstarch
- ½ cup water
- 1 tsp. sea salt
- 1 tsp. freshly ground pepper

1. Heat the oil in a skillet over medium-high heat. Add the meat strips in batches and cook each batch for 3 to 4 minutes, or until browned. Add the onions and sauté for 2 to 3 more minutes. Add the garlic, mushrooms, and carrots and stir-fry for 2 to 3 more minutes, or until the carrots begin to soften. Stir in the stock, Worcestershire sauce, and dill. Reduce the heat to low, cover, and cook, stirring occasionally, for 15 minutes.

2. Place the cornstarch, water, salt, and pepper in a small bowl and stir until smooth. Pour the cornstarch slurry into the stroganoff mixture. Bring the liquid to a boil and stir until the sauce has thickened. Stir in sour cream or cream cheese and heat through, but do not allow to boil.

3. Serve with noodles, rice, or potatoes. Serves 4.

* Worcestershire sauce contains anchovies, so it's not vegetarian.

** The last time I prepared Beef Stroganoff, I realized I didn't have sour cream in the fridge. I remembered that my friends Tara and Val had invited me to dinner at their house a while back and they'd substituted cream cheese for the sour cream in the dish they'd served me. I happened to have some cream cheese, so I used it instead. It changed the stroganoff from "really good" to "awesome and company-worthy."

Spinach and Sun-Dried Tomato-Stuffed Steak

Yum! Sun-dried tomatoes! They pack a flavourful punch. To save on calories or fat, choose sun-dried tomatoes that are not packed in oil—just make sure you soften them in a little hot water before using them.

- **1½ to 2 lbs. lean sirloin beef steak**
- **sea salt to taste**
- **freshly ground pepper to taste**
- **1 (10 oz.) package frozen chopped spinach, thawed and well drained**
- **⅓ cup sun-dried tomatoes, sliced into small pieces**
- **2 tbsp. grated Parmesan cheese**
- **2 tbsp. chopped fresh basil**

1. Preheat the grill or barbecue to medium or turn on the broiler of the oven.

2. Score the meat by making shallow diagonal cuts at 1-inch intervals in a diamond pattern on both sides. Place the meat on a chopping block between 2 pieces of plastic wrap. Working from the centre to the edges, pound it into a rectangle shape using the flat side of a meat mallet. Remove the plastic wrap and sprinkle with salt and pepper.

3. Spread the spinach over the steak in an even layer. Sprinkle the sun-dried tomatoes, Parmesan cheese, and basil evenly over the top.

4. Roll the steak up from the short side. Secure the roll with wooden toothpicks or metal skewers at 1½-inch intervals. Brush the roll liberally with the reserved marinade.

5. If cooking on a grill or barbecue, place the roll directly on the grill. If cooking in the oven, place the meat on a broiler pan 3 to 4 inches from the top element. Cook to desired doneness*, turning once.

6. Remove the skewers or toothpicks, slice, and serve. Serves 4.

*Allow 10 to 12 minutes for medium-rare, and 12 to 16 minutes for medium.

Treats and Sweets

This chapter has a little of everything. We have some healthier vegan choices, such as Spelt, Cranberry, and Walnut Crumb Cake *(page 186)*, Cornmeal Muffins *(page 182)*, and Tofu Cheesecake *(page 189)*. We have the much-sought-after recipe for my famous biscuits. And then we have out-of-the-ordinary choices like Tasty Tahini Carrot Cake *(page 195)* and Ginger, Orange, and Thyme Loaf *(page 196)*. I also had to include the butter-laden, sugary special-occasion desserts that you really want the recipe for, including "How to Get Invited to a Christmas Party" Squares *(page 170)*, Boterkoek (Dutch Butter Cake - *page 200*), and Speculaas (Dutch Spice Cake - *page 201*).

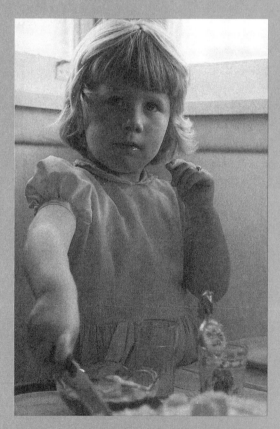

This is me at age 4 helping my mom out in the kitchen (most likely making sweets)

Cornmeal Muffins

vegan

We served these muffins at the farmers' market with our Southwest Tofu Scramble (page 89) or our Soup of the Day.

- 1 cup unsweetened soy milk
- 1 tsp. cider vinegar
- 1 cup organic stone-ground cornmeal
- 1 cup whole wheat or spelt flour
- ⅛ cup sugar
- 1 tsp. baking powder
- ½ tsp. sea salt
- ¼ cup oil
- 1 cup fresh or frozen corn kernels

1. Preheat the oven to 350°F.

2. Combine the soy milk and cider vinegar in a small mixing bowl.

3. Combine the cornmeal, flour, sugar, baking powder, and salt in a large mixing bowl. Add the soy milk mixture, the oil, and the corn. Mix gently, taking care not to overwork the mix.

4. Divide the mixture evenly into a lightly greased 12-cup muffin tin. Bake in the preheated oven for 25 to 30 minutes, or until a toothpick inserted into the centre comes out clean. Makes 12 muffins.

Karin's Coveted Biscuits

vegetarian

Many people have asked for this recipe, but few have received it. Here is your chance.

- 1½ cups whole wheat flour
- 1½ cups unbleached white flour
- ¼ cup sugar
- 1 tbsp. baking powder
- 1 tsp. baking soda
- 1 tsp. sea salt
- 2 tsp. cream of tartar
- ¾ cup chilled butter
- 1 cup milk

1. Preheat the oven to 425°F.

2. Combine the whole wheat and white flours, sugar, baking powder, baking soda, sea salt, and cream of tartar in a large mixing bowl. Use a pastry cutter to cut in the butter until the butter chunks are as small as peas. Stir in the milk with a fork. Continue to stir just until the mixture forms a soft dough.

3. Knead the dough 6 to 8 times, or until the ingredients are combined. For tender and fluffy biscuits, you don't want to over work the dough. Drop the dough by tablespoons onto an ungreased baking sheet about 1½ inches apart. Bake for 10 to 12 minutes. Makes 20 to 24 biscuits.

Nice Buns

vegetarian with vegan option

Impress your friends at the next barbecue with these golden-brown rolls, which are light and tender and simple to prepare. If you are wanting "Nice Vegan Buns" instead, use soy milk or almond milk.

- **1 cup milk, soy milk, or almond milk**
- **¾ cup water**
- **½ cup vegetable oil**
- **¼ cup white sugar**
- **1 teaspoon salt**
- **4 to 5 cups all-purpose flour, divided**
- **2 tbsp. dry yeast**

1. In a small pot over low heat, combine the milk, water, oil, sugar, and salt. Heat to lukewarm, about 100°F.

2. In a large bowl, combine 2 cups of the flour with the yeast. Add the heated milk mixture and beat until smooth, about 3 minutes.

3. Mix in the remaining 2 to 3 cups of flour a little at a time until a soft dough has formed. Turn the dough out onto a floured surface, cover it with an upside-down bowl, and let it rest for about 10 minutes.

4. Shape the dough into 12 slightly flat balls, or whatever shape you like. Place the dough balls on a greased baking sheet in a warm area and let them rise for 1½ to 2 hours, or until they have doubled in size.

5. Preheat the oven to 400°F.

6. Bake in the preheated oven for 12 to 15 minutes, or until the tops are golden brown. Makes 12 buns.

Pizza Cookies

vegetarian

Healthy savoury cookies! Try these if you are watching your sugar intake. If you want to be flexible and adventurous, use whatever ingredients you have in your fridge to make your own pizza cookies. How about some chopped bell peppers? Or jalapeños, if you like a little heat?

- 1½ cups unbleached white flour
- 1 cup whole wheat flour
- 2 tsp. baking powder
- ½ tsp. baking soda
- ½ tsp. sea salt
- 1 tsp. dried basil
- ½ tsp. dried oregano
- 1 tsp. freshly ground pepper
- 5 sun-dried tomatoes, finely chopped
- 2½ cups shredded cheese (your choice), divided
- 4 green onions, sliced thin
- 1 egg
- 1⅓ cups buttermilk or sour milk
- ⅓ cup vegetable oil
- 2 cloves garlic, minced

1. Preheat the oven to 375°F.

2. Combine the white and whole wheat flours, baking powder, baking soda, sea salt, basil, oregano, and pepper in a large mixing bowl. Stir in the sun-dried tomatoes, any other vegetables you wish to use, 1½ cups of the cheese, and the green onions.

3. Whisk the egg in another medium-sized mixing bowl. Add the buttermilk, oil, and garlic and whisk to combine.

4. Pour the egg mixture into the flour mixture and stir until combined. Drop the dough by tablespoons onto a lightly greased baking sheet about 1 inch apart. Sprinkle the cookies with the remaining cheese. Bake in the preheated oven for 12 to 15 minutes, or until the cheese is melted and golden brown. Makes 12 to 15 large cookies.

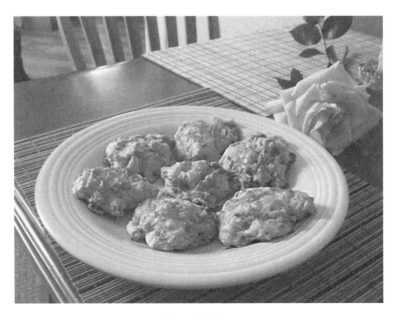

Pizza Cookies

Herb and Cheese Zucchini Bread

vegetarian

Zucchini bread is popular during the harvest season when everyone has way too many zucchinis to use up. This dish reminds me of one particular day during the harvest, when I was buying zucchini at the farmers' market for the catering business. Someone came along, saw all the zucchinis in my basket, and asked, "Don't you have any friends?" That's just what it is like here in Charlottetown. I've heard of people waking up and finding baskets of zucchinis on their doorstep.

This recipe is for a savoury loaf. Try it; it may be your new favourite.

- 1 cup unbleached white flour
- 1 cup whole wheat flour
- 2 tsp. baking powder
- ½ tsp. baking soda
- ¾ tsp. sea salt
- ¼ tsp. freshly ground pepper
- pinch cayenne pepper
- 2 tbsp. of your favourite chopped fresh herbs (dill, parsley, rosemary, basil, oregano, etc.)
- 2 tbsp. finely chopped green onions
- 1½ cup your choice grated cheese (cheddar, mozzarella, goat cheese, Parmesan, Asiago, or a combination), divided
- 2 eggs
- ¼ cup olive oil
- ½ cup milk
- 1 cup shredded zucchini

1. Preheat the oven to 350°F.

2. Combine white and whole wheat flour, baking powder, baking soda, salt, pepper, cayenne, herbs, green onions, and all but 2 tablespoons of the cheese in a large mixing bowl.

3. In a separate medium-sized bowl, beat the eggs lightly. Add the olive oil and milk and mix well. Stir in the zucchini.

4. Add the liquid mixture to the flour mixture and stir just until all the dry ingredients are moistened. Do not overmix.

5. Pour the batter into a lightly greased loaf pan, and smooth the top. Sprinkle with the remaining 2 tablespoons of cheese. Bake in the preheated oven for 40 to 45 minutes, or until a toothpick inserted in the centre comes out clean.

6. Let the loaf stand for 15 minutes, then turn it out onto a wire rack and allow it to cool completely before eating. Makes 1 large loaf or 2 small loaves. Serves 6 to 8.

Spelt, Cranberry, and Walnut Crumb Cake, a.k.a. Catch (or Keep) a Husband Cake

vegan

I have deep suspicions that my husband married me to get this cake. I still make sure I make this for him often. We sold out of this cake almost every week at the farmers' market.

- ⅓ (420 g) package soft tofu
- 1 cup soy milk
- 1 tbsp. apple cider vinegar
- 2½ cups spelt flour
- 1 cup organic cane sugar
- 3 tsp. ground cinnamon
- 1 tsp. ground ginger
- ½ tsp. salt
- ¾ cup vegetable oil
- 1 tsp. baking powder
- 1 tsp. baking soda
- 1½ cups dried cranberries, divided
- 1 cup walnut crumbs

1. Preheat the oven to 350°F.

2. Place the tofu and soy milk in the bowl of a food processor and blend to combine. Add the apple cider vinegar. Set aside.

3. Combine the flour, sugar, cinnamon, ginger, salt, and vegetable oil in a large mixing bowl. Remove 1 cup of the mixture, place it in another small bowl, and set aside.

4. Pulse the mixture in the food processor again. If there is room in the processor, add the contents of the large bowl, along with the baking powder and baking soda, and process until smooth. If there isn't enough room in the food processor for all of the ingredients, add the contents of the processor, the baking soda, and the powder to the large bowl and mix well. Add ¾ cup of the dried cranberries and mix to combine.

5. Spread the batter into a lightly greased 9" × 13" baking dish.

6. Add the walnuts and remaining ¾ cup of cranberries to the remaining 1 cup of flour mixture and stir to combine. Spread the flour mixture evenly on top of the batter.

7. Bake in the preheated oven for 30 to 40 minutes, or until the cake feels firm to the touch. Serves 12 people (or one hungry husband!).

Mike loves this cake so much that he proposed to me on top of the Eiffel Tower. We were married the next year on a beach in PEI.

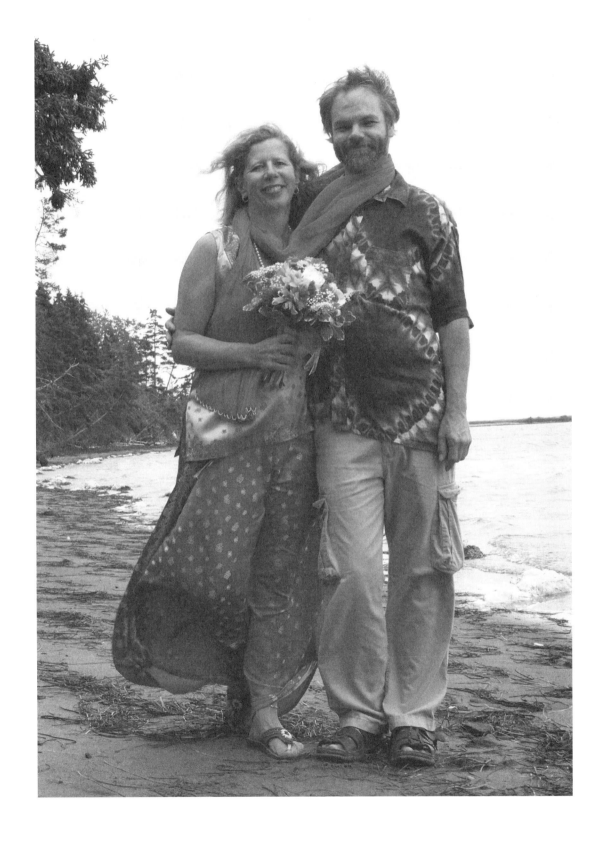

Vegan Coconut Cake

vegan
gluten-free option

It was a blessed day for me when Margaret came to work in the Eat Well kitchen. We became very good friends and excellent travel buddies. This light and delicious cake comes from Margaret's collection. She brought it to a potluck and I couldn't stay away from it. I begged her to share it with you, and so she did.

- 1 ⅔ cups cane sugar
- ⅔ cup coconut oil
- 1 (14 oz.) can coconut milk
- ¼ cup almond milk
- ¼ cup lemon juice
- zest of 1 lemon
- 2 tsp. vanilla
- 1 ½ cups whole wheat or quinoa flour
- 1 ½ cups coconut flour
- 2 tsp. baking powder
- 1 tsp. baking soda
- 1 tsp. sea salt
- 1 ½ cups unsweetened shredded coconut

1. Preheat the oven to 350°F.

2. Combine the sugar, coconut oil, coconut milk, almond milk, lemon juice, lemon zest, and vanilla in a large mixing bowl or food processor.

3. In a separate large bowl, combine the whole wheat or quinoa flour, coconut flour, baking powder, baking soda, and salt.

4. Blend the flour mixture into the wet mixture in batches, stirring or processing well after each addition. Fold in the shredded coconut.

5. Pour the batter into a lightly greased and floured 8- or 10-inch Bundt or cheesecake pan. Bake for 1 hour, or until a knife inserted into the centre comes out clean.

6. Allow the cake to cool for about 10 minutes in the pan. Run a knife around the edge of the pan, and then turn the pan upside down to release the cake. Serves 8 to 10.

Margaret and me exploring the cuisine in Paris
(our favourite hobby in any country!).

Tofu Cheesecake

vegan

I've tried many recipes for tofu cheesecake, and this one is the winner. You can also make this a savoury cheesecake—just replace the graham cracker crumbs with any savoury cracker crumb, switch the honey and vanilla with herbs and garlic or pesto, and garnish with roasted or sautéed vegetables.

- **2 (4 oz.) packages graham crackers**
- **¾ cup vegan margarine, softened**
- **1 tbsp. cornstarch**
- **2 tbsp. water**
- **2 lbs. firm tofu, cubed**
- **½ tsp. salt**
- **¼ cup lemon juice**
- **½ cup mild-flavoured oil**
- **½ cup honey**
- **2 tsp. vanilla**
- **your favourite fruit for garnish**

1. Preheat the oven to 350°F.

2. Place the crackers in the bowl of a food processor and process until they form fine crumbs. Add the margarine and process until combined. Press the cracker mixture firmly into the bottom of a lightly greased 9-inch springform pan. Set aside.

3. In a small bowl, mix the cornstarch with the water until dissolved. Place the cornstarch mixture, tofu, salt, lemon juice, oil, honey, and vanilla in a clean food processor bowl and blend for 2 to 3 minutes, or until creamy.

4. Pour the tofu mixture into the crust. Bake in the preheated oven for 40 minutes, or until the cake is firm and the top is golden brown. Serves 8 to 10.

5. Chill and garnish with fruit before serving.

Vegan Wacky or Mexican Wackier Cake

vegan
gluten-free option

Do you remember having this cake when you were young(er)? It is a great one! You mix and bake it in one pan. It contains no animal products, and you can also make it gluten-free by using gluten-free flour mix instead of all-purpose flour. Switch it up and call it a Mexican Wackier Cake by adding 2 teaspoons of ground cinnamon and ¼ teaspoon of chili powder to the dry mix.

- **1 ½ cups all-purpose flour or gluten-free flour mix***
- **1 cup cane sugar**
- **½ tsp. salt**
- **1 tsp. baking soda**
- **¼ cup plus 3 tbsp. unsweetened cocoa powder, divided**
- **1 tsp. vanilla**
- **1 tbsp. cider vinegar**
- **5 tbsp. sunflower oil**
- **1 ¼ cup warm water, divided**
- **1 cup icing sugar, sifted**

1. Preheat the oven to 350°F.

2. Sift the flour, sugar, salt, baking soda, and 3 tablespoons of the cocoa powder together into an ungreased 8" × 8" cake pan.

3. Make three large depressions in the flour mixture. Pour the vanilla into one well, the vinegar into the second, and oil into the third. Pour 1 cup of the water over everything, and stir well with fork.

4. Bake in the preheated oven for 30 to 40 minutes, or until a toothpick inserted into the centre comes out clean.

5. While the cake is baking, combine the icing sugar and the remaining ¼ cup of cocoa powder together in a medium-sized mixing bowl. Stir in 1 tablespoon of the remaining ¼ cup of water at a time until the mixture is thin enough to pour. Pour the chocolate glaze evenly over the warm cake, let cool for 30 minutes, and serve. Serves 4 to 6.

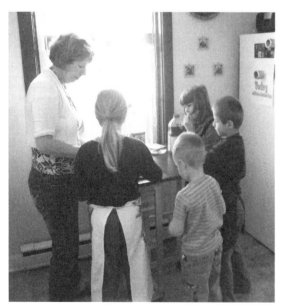

My precious nieces and nephews getting a cooking lesson.

*For the gluten-free flour mix, combine 3 cups of white rice flour with 1 cup of potato starch and ½ cup of tapioca starch. Store the extra flour in an air-tight container for next time you make this dish.

Vegan Chocolate Mousse

vegan
gluten-free

Isn't it great to know that even when you are on a vegan and/or gluten-free diet, you can still enjoy delicious and decadent treats such as this Chocolate Mousse?

- **1 lb. (approx. 2 cups) soft tofu, rinsed and drained**
- **2 tbsp. mild-flavoured oil**
- **1 tbsp. almond butter or tahini**
- **6 tbsp. brown sugar**
- **1 cup vegan chocolate chips, melted**
- **5 tbsp. cocoa powder**
- **⅓ cup maple syrup**
- **1 tsp. vanilla**
- **Pecan Praline (page 192) for garnish**

1. Place all of the ingredients in the bowl of a food processor and blend, scraping the sides of the bowl with a spatula periodically, until smooth and creamy.

2. Divide the mixture evenly among 4 to 6 parfait glasses. Chill in the refrigerator for at least 30 minutes before serving. Garnish with Pecan Praline (page 192) before serving. Serves 4 to 6.

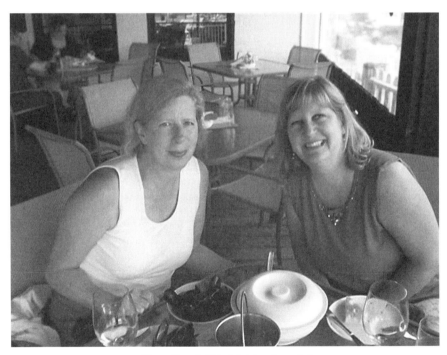

Nancy Russell. This dish is her favourite!

Pecan Praline

vegan
gluten-free

Here is a nice vegan treat you can serve during Christmas or any other special occasion. Or try crumbling it and serving it on top of our Vegan Chocolate Mousse (page 191).

- ¾ cups turbinado sugar
- ⅓ cup light brown sugar
- ⅓ cup soy milk
- 2 tbsp. vegan margarine
- 1 cup pecans
- ½ tsp. vanilla

1. Combine the turbinado and light brown sugars, soy milk, and vegan margarine in a heavy pan over medium-high heat. Stir constantly until the mixture starts to boil. Reduce the heat to low and simmer, stirring constantly, until the mixture reaches soft ball stage, or 235°F.

2. Remove the mixture from the heat, add the vanilla and pecans, and stir for 3 to 5 minutes, or until the batter gets very creamy and cloudy. Once the mixture is cloudy, pour it onto a large sheet of wax paper and spread it out with a spatula. (If it is too thick to pour, stir in a tablespoon of warm soy milk.) Set it aside to cool. Once it has hardened, break it into pieces and store it in a sealed container. Makes ¾ cup to 1 cup.

Vegan Chocolate Chip Cookies

vegan

This was one of my favourite treats while I was on a vegan diet.

- 1 cup vegan margarine
- 1 cup cane sugar
- 2 tbsp. molasses
- ¼ cup soft or silken tofu
- 1 tsp. vanilla extract
- 1 cup whole wheat flour
- 1 cup unbleached white flour
- ½ tsp. baking soda
- ¼ tsp. sea salt
- 2 cups vegan chocolate chips
- ½ cup walnut pieces*

1. In a large mixing bowl, cream the margarine, sugar, and molasses together until light and fluffy. Add the tofu and vanilla and beat until well blended.

2. In a separate medium-sized mixing bowl, combine the whole wheat and white flours, baking soda, and salt. Add the dry mixture to the wet mixture and stir well to combine. Stir in the chocolate chips and walnuts.

3. Drop the batter by teaspoonfuls about an inch apart onto an ungreased baking sheet. Bake in the preheated oven for 8 to 10 minutes, or until golden brown. Makes about 5 dozen cookies.

*Optional

Hearty Himalayan Rice Pudding

vegan
gluten-free

This nicely spiced pudding is vegan, gluten-free, and made with whole grains. After eating a bowl of this, you will be able to climb mountains. You can also switch this recipe up by replacing the apricots, raisins, and dates with your own choice of fruit, such as coconut, cranberries, currants, dried apple, or figs.

- **1 cup uncooked brown rice**
- **2 cups water**
- **1 cup apple cider or apple juice**
- **1 whole cinnamon stick
  or 2 tsp. ground cinnamon**
- **1 tsp. cardamom powder**
- **¼ tsp. ground cloves**
- **½ tsp. sea salt**
- **2 cups soy milk**
- **¼ cup diced dried apricots**
- **¼ cup Thompson raisins**
- **½ cup brown rice syrup or maple syrup**
- **¼ cup diced dried, pitted dates**
- **½ cup toasted and chopped nuts (your choice)**

1. Place the brown rice and water in a medium-sized saucepan over high heat and bring to a boil. Reduce the heat to low, cover, and cook the rice for 45 minutes.

2. Stir in the apple cider or juice, cinnamon, cardamom, cloves, sea salt, soy milk, apricots, and raisins and cook for another 15 minutes, stirring occasionally. Add the syrup, dates, and nuts and cook for another 5 minutes.

3. Adjust the sweetness to taste by adding extra syrup if needed. Serves 6 to 8.

Freakin' Good Flourless Chocolate Cake

gluten-free

Do you have a guest with a gluten-free diet? Don't panic, here is the answer to your dessert dilemma.

A food processor makes this recipe "a piece of cake" to make.

- **16 oz. dark chocolate**
- **1 cup light brown sugar, packed**
- **½ cup white sugar**
- **¾ cup very hot strong coffee**
- **1 cup room-temperature butter, cut into pieces**
- **2 tbsp. unsweetened cocoa powder**
- **8 room-temperature eggs**
- **1 tbsp. vanilla extract**
- **chocolate sauce for garnish**
- **powdered sugar for garnish**
- **berries or mint leaves for garnish**

1. Preheat the oven to 350°F.

2. Break the dark chocolate up into pieces and place them in the bowl of a food processor. Pulse until the chocolate breaks up into small bits. Add the brown and white sugars and pulse until the chocolate and sugar turn into an even, sandy grain. Pour the coffee slowly into the feed tube as you pulse again. Pulse until the chocolate is melted.

3. Add the butter pieces and the cocoa powder, and pulse to combine. Next add the eggs and vanilla, and process until smooth, liquid, and creamy.

4. Wrap the bottom and sides of a lightly greased 10-cup springform pan with foil. Pour the batter into the pan.

5. Bake in the centre of the preheated oven for 55 to 65 minutes, or until puffed and cracked and a wooden toothpick comes out clean.

6. Place the cake pan on a wire rack to cool. The cake will deflate. When partially cooled, press down on it gently with a spatula to make it even.

7. Once the cake has cooled completely, cover it with foil or plastic wrap and chill it in the refrigerator for at least three hours or overnight. To garnish, drizzle with chocolate sauce and/or sprinkle with powdered sugar and top with berries and/or mint leaves. Serves 8 to 10.

Tasty Tahini Carrot Cake

vegetarian

This is a different but delicious spin on carrot cake—there is tahini in the cake and also in the topping. I've taken this cake to many events and received plenty of compliments and pleas for the recipe.

- 1¼ cups tahini, divided
- ¾ cup vegetable oil
- 1½ cup unbleached white flour
- 1 tsp. vanilla
- 1 tsp. ground allspice
- 4 eggs
- 1½ cups brown sugar
- 1 tsp. ground cinnamon
- 1 tsp. salt
- 1 tsp. baking soda
- 1 tsp. baking powder
- 1 cup chopped walnuts
- 3 cups unpeeled, scrubbed, and grated carrots
- ½ cup honey

1. Preheat the oven to 350°F.

2. Combine ¾ cup of the tahini, the vegetable oil, flour, vanilla, allspice, eggs, brown sugar, cinnamon, salt, baking soda, baking powder, and walnuts in a large bowl. Add the carrots and stir well.

3. Pour the batter into a lightly greased Bundt pan or 10-inch springform pan. Bake for 1 hour and 15 minutes or until a toothpick inserted into the centre comes out clean. Cool and invert onto a cake plate.

4. Combine the remaining ½ cup of tahini with the honey and mix well. Pour the mixture evenly over the cake and serve. Serves 8 to 10.

Ginger, Orange, and Thyme Loaf

vegetarian

I saw this recipe in the newspaper long ago and the ingredients looked unusual enough to capture my attention. The ginger, orange, and thyme make up a very nice flavour and I'm betting no one else will be bringing this to the potluck.

- 1 cup soft butter
- 2 cups sugar, divided
- 1 tbsp. grated orange zest
- 1½ tsp. chopped fresh thyme, divided
- 5 eggs
- 2 tsp. vanilla
- 2 cups unbleached white flour
- 1 tsp. ground ginger
- 1 tsp. sea salt
- ½ cup plus 2 tbsp. finely chopped candied ginger, divided
- ¼ cup orange juice

1. Preheat the oven to 350°F.

2. Place the butter in a large mixing bowl and blend it with a hand mixer until it is very soft. Slowly add 1¾ cups of the sugar, continuing to beat until the mixture is light and fluffy.

3. Mix in the orange zest and the 1 teaspoon of the thyme. Add the eggs one at time while continuing to beat the mixture. Mix in the vanilla.

4. In a separate medium-sized mixing bowl, combine the flour, ground ginger, and salt. Add the flour mixture to the liquid mixture and beat until just incorporated. Fold in ½ cup of the candied ginger.

5. Pour into a lightly greased loaf pan and bake for 60 to 70 minutes, or until a toothpick inserted into the centre comes out clean. Allow to cool.

6. While the cake is cooling, combine the remaining ¼ cup of sugar, the orange juice, and the remaining ½ teaspoon of thyme in a pot over medium heat. Bring to a boil and reduce for 1 to 2 minutes, or until the syrup is slightly thickened.

7. Poke holes in the cooled loaf with a wooden skewer. Brush the syrup over the cake, letting it soak into the holes. Sprinkle the remaining candied ginger on top and serve. Serves 6 to 8.

Survivor Cookies

vegetarian

If you were stranded on a desert island with only a sealed container of these cookies, they may save your life. How, you ask? Well, as soon as you open the container, someone is sure to come along and ask you to share.

Remember that even though this recipe calls for a lot of butter, it makes a very large batch. These cookies were a favourite for catering functions. I would pre-roll some raw cookies and freeze them so I could just pop a few in the oven for fresh cookies anytime.

- **2 cups butter**
- **1¼ cups white sugar**
- **1½ cups brown sugar**
- **3 eggs**
- **2½ cups flour**
- **1¼ tsp. baking soda**
- **½ tsp. salt**
- **3¾ cups rolled oats**
- **¾ cup poppy seeds**
- **1½ cups sunflower seeds**
- **1½ cups pumpkin seeds**
- **2½ cups chopped dates or chocolate chips**
- **1 tbsp. vanilla**

1. Preheat the oven to 350°F.

2. Cream the butter in a large mixing bowl. Mix in the white and brown sugar. Add the eggs one at a time, stirring to combine after each egg is added.

3. In a separate large mixing bowl, combine the flour, baking soda, salt, rolled oats, poppy seeds, sunflower seeds, and pumpkin seeds. Gradually add the flour mixture to the butter, sugar, and egg mixture, stirring constantly. Stir in the dates or chocolate chips and vanilla.

4. Drop the batter by teaspoonfuls onto a greased baking sheet about an inch apart. Bake in the preheated oven for 12 to 15 minutes, or until golden brown. Makes about 8 dozen cookies.

Mrs. Hennessey's Aunt Jean's Chocolate Chip Cookies

vegetarian

I never met Aunt Jean, but it was Mrs. Hennessey, a lady I worked with, who gave us this recipe when my children were very young. This has been made at least 400 times in our house. It makes a good, large batch so we usually freeze a few—but not for long!

- 1½ cups shortening
- 3 cups brown sugar
- 4 eggs
- 4 cups unbleached white flour, divided
- 2 tsp. baking soda
- 2 tsp. baking powder
- 2 tsp. salt
- 3 tsp. vanilla
- 2 cups chocolate chips
- ½ cup crushed nuts*

*Optional

1. Preheat the oven to 350°F.

2. Place the shortening and brown sugar in a large mixing bowl and cream them together with a hand blender. Add the eggs one at a time, mixing constantly. Blend in the vanilla.

3. In a large bowl, combine 3½ cups of the flour with the baking soda, baking powder, and salt. Slowly add the flour mixture to the shortening mixture, and then stir in the remaining ½ cup of flour. Fold in the chocolate chips and nuts.

4. Drop teaspoon-sized dollops of the dough onto a lightly greased baking sheet about 1 inch apart. Bake for 8 to 10 minutes, or until the cookies are lightly browned. Makes about 6 dozen.

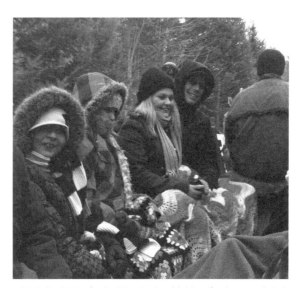

My son Ken is the cookie baker in the family. Here he is with his wife, Anna, and their two lovely children.

"How to Get Invited to a Christmas Party" Squares

vegetarian

I've been asked many times to share this recipe, but I was worried that if I did, I would never get invited to another Christmas party! It's time to let go.

- 1¾ cup **Oreo** cookie crumbs
- ½ cup melted butter
- 1 (300 ml) can sweetened condensed milk
- 2 cups chopped white chocolate
- 1½ cups dried cranberries
- 1 cup toasted coconut
- 1 cup pecan pieces

1. Preheat the oven to 350°F.

2. Combine the cookie crumbs and butter in a medium-sized mixing bowl. Press the crumb mixture firmly into the bottom of a square 9-inch pan.

3. Combine the condensed milk, white chocolate, cranberries, toasted coconut, and pecans in a large mixing bowl. Pour the mixture over the crumb base and spread it evenly over the top.

4. Bake for 25 to 30 minutes, stirring it once halfway through the cooking time to spread the white chocolate around. Cool and slice into small squares. Makes about 24 squares.

Boterkoek (Dutch Butter Cake)

vegetarian

This is usually a Christmas treat, but we would make it on other special occasions as well. My brothers loved to come home for the holidays just so they could get this treat.

- **1 cup butter**
- **1 cup sugar**
- **2 cups flour**
- **½ tsp. salt**
- **½ tsp. almond extract**
- **1 beaten egg, divided**
- **slivered almonds for garnish**

1. Preheat the oven to 350°F.

2. In a large mixing bowl, combine the butter and sugar. Add the flour, salt, almond extract, and all but 1 tablespoon of the beaten egg and knead into a firm ball.

3. Press the dough into a greased 8" × 8" baking pan. Brush the top with the reserved tablespoon of beaten egg. Add the slivered almonds on top for decoration.

4. Bake in the preheated oven for 30 minutes, or until golden brown. Cool and slice into squares before serving. Makes about 16 squares.

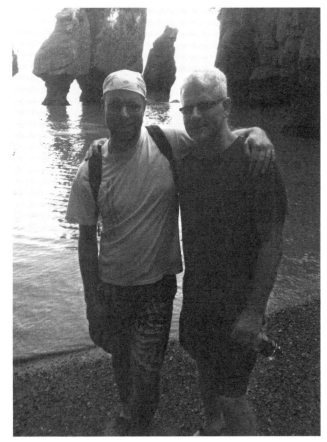

My brothers—the best ones ever! Jeff Zaat on the left and Steve Zaat on the right.

Speculaas (Dutch Spice Cake)

vegetarian

This is a special treat that we would have around Christmas. This recipe came from my mom. I can still hear her voice when I read it. She would be very happy that I am sharing her recipe with you. "Eet smakelijk!" ("Eat yummy!" in Dutch).

- **I cup white sugar, divided**
- **¾ cup brown sugar**
- **2 cups flour**
- **½ tsp. sea salt**
- **I tsp. baking soda**
- **I tbsp. speculaas spice mix***
- **I cup chilled butter**
- **5 tbsp. milk**
- **2 cups almonds**
- **I beaten egg, divided**
- **zest of ½ lemon**
- **slivered almonds for garnish**

1. Combine ¾ cup of the white sugar with the brown sugar, flour, salt, baking soda, and spice mix in a large mixing bowl. Cut in the chilled butter. Add the milk I tablespoon at a time, stirring constantly, until the dough is moist enough to knead into a ball. Cover with plastic wrap and place in the refrigerator to chill for I hour.

2. While the dough is chilling, place the almonds in the bowl of a food processor and process until ground. Add the remaining ¼ cup of sugar, all but I tablespoon of the egg, and lemon zest and process until combined.

3. Preheat the oven to 350°F.

4. Remove the chilled dough from the fridge and divide it into two equal pieces. Press one piece of the dough into the bottom of a greased 8-inch square pan. Spread the almond paste evenly over the dough in the pan. Press the other half of the dough on top. Brush the reserved tablespoon of egg over the top. Sprinkle the slivered almonds on top for decoration.

5. Bake in the preheated oven for 45 to 55 minutes, or until golden brown and a toothpick inserted in the centre comes out clean.

6. Remove from the pan and cool on a wire rack. Cut into wedges or diamonds before serving. Serves 8 to 10.

*To make the speculaas spice mix, combine 2 tbsp. ground cinnamon, I tsp. ground ginger, ¼ tsp. ground nutmeg, ¼ tsp. cardamom powder, ¼ tsp. cloves, ¼ tsp. ground anise, and ¼ tsp. freshly ground pepper. Store the leftover spice mix in an air-tight container for next time you make these squares.

Sticky Date Pudding with Toffee Sauce

vegetarian

This is the most requested of all my recipes. At Christmas time I would make 30 to 40 of these in the Eat Well kitchen for families who made this their annual tradition.

- **2 cups water**
- **½ cups chopped dates**
- **4 tsp. baking soda**
- **1 cup white sugar**
- **⅓ cup butter, softened**
- **3 eggs**
- **2 cups white flour**
- **1 tbsp. baking powder**
- **½ tsp. ground ginger**

1. Preheat the oven to 350°F.

2. Bring the water and dates to a boil in a medium saucepan over high heat. Reduce the heat to low and cook until the dates are soft, about 5 minutes. Remove from heat and carefully add the baking soda (it will foam up). Set aside to cool.

3. In a large bowl, beat the sugar and butter together with an electric mixer until light. Add the eggs and beat until combined.

4. In a separate medium-sized mixing bowl, whisk together the flour, baking powder, and ginger. Add the flour mixture and the date mixture to the butter and sugar mixture in small batches, alternating between the two. Mix until well blended.

5. Pour the batter into a greased 9-inch square pan. Set the square pan in a larger shallow pan and pour hot water into the larger pan until it comes 1 inch up the side of the smaller pan. Bake in centre of the preheated oven for 50 minutes, or until a toothpick inserted in the centre comes out clean. Serve with Toffee Sauce (recipe below). Serves 6.

Toffee Sauce

This toffee sauce is the best! Like my friend Tara says, "the cake is merely a vehicle to get the toffee sauce to your mouth."

- **¾ cup butter**
- **1¼ cups packed brown sugar**
- **¾ cup whipping cream**
- **½ teaspoon vanilla**

1. Melt the butter in a medium-sized saucepan over medium heat. Add the brown sugar and stir until dissolved. Add the cream and bring to simmer, stirring occasionally, until slightly thickened. Stir in the vanilla. Serve warm with Sticky Date Pudding. Makes about 1½ cups to 2 cups.

Gluten-Free Shortbread Cookies

gluten-free

Here is a recipe for tasty shortbread cookies without gluten. You can also spice them up with the suggested variations below.

This mix also works as a gluten-free pie or cheesecake crust. Just press the dough into the base of a springform pan or pie plate and bake for about 10 to 12 minutes.

- **½ cup almond flour**
- **½ cup rice flour**
- **½ cup cornstarch**
- **½ cup icing sugar**
- **½ cup butter, cut into pieces**

1. Sift the almond flour, rice flour, cornstarch, and icing sugar together in a large bowl. Add the butter and, using a pastry blender, cut until you get a crumbly dough. Using your hands, mix until a soft dough forms. Do not overmix.

2. Cover the dough in plastic wrap and refrigerate for 1 hour.

3. Preheat the oven to 325°F.

4. Divide and shape the chilled dough into 1-inch balls. Place the dough balls about 1 inch apart on a greased cookie sheet and flatten them with a lightly floured fork.

5. Bake in the preheated oven for 15 to 20 minutes, or until the edges are lightly browned. Makes about 4 dozen cookies.

Suggested Variations

- Mix 2 tablespoons of finely chopped lemon or orange peel into the dough before chilling.

- Mix 2 tablespoons of finely chopped nuts into the dough before chilling.

- Mix 1 teaspoon of coconut extract and 2 tablespoons of grated lime zest into the dough before chilling.

- Mix 2 tablespoons of chopped walnuts and 1 teaspoon of minced fresh rosemary into the dough before chilling.

- Mix 2 tablespoons of finely chopped lemon peel and 1 tablespoon of lavender into the dough before chilling.

- Make chai shortbreads by mixing 2 teaspoons ground ginger, 1 teaspoon ground cinnamon, ½ teaspoon cardamom powder, ½ teaspoon ground nutmeg, and ¼ teaspoon cloves into the dough before chilling.

- Before baking, make deep thumbprints in the cookies and fill with your favourite preserves.

- Once baked and cooled, dip the cookies into melted chocolate.

- Once baked and cooled, top the cookies with a glaze made with 1 cup powdered sugar, 2 teaspoons vanilla, and 1 to 2 teaspoons water.

Martini Monday

After I was diagnosed with untreatable cancer and I sold my business, I was missing my friends. So a group of my girlfriends and I decided to start a club. We called it "Martini Monday."

Every second Monday, we would go to one of the girls' houses (usually Lori's). One girl would make the drinks, two girls would bring food for snacking, and we would all play a game. Everyone would throw in $5 to pay for the drinks.

Only once did we ever have a real martini, but it wasn't too popular, so we didn't try that again. Instead we would take any cocktail recipe, multiply it by ten to make a pitcher full, and pour it into martini glasses.

These evenings were so great and healing. We'd have a lot of laughter, some tears, tons of support, and always a wonderful feeling of sisterhood.

I felt that this book should end on a fun note, with the Martini Monday story and some of our concoctions/recipes. These recipes are all for a single serving. Feel free to do as the Martini Monday ladies do and use a calculator (or guess) to make a pitcher full.

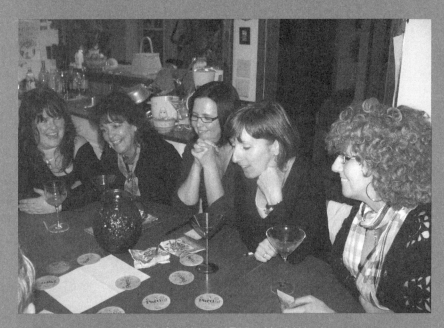

Lori, Sylvie, Sue, Nora and Trish at Martini Monday

The Cosmopolitan Martini

This was the very first Martini Monday recipe and the inspiration that started it all. My friend Julia Sauve, who is a New York native, and I took a road trip to New York City to cross an entry off my bucket list. It was a dream come true for me. Julia and I went to Grand Central Station on a Monday evening and there was a sign at the bar that said "Martini Monday."

- **½ oz. Cointreau or orange liqueur**
- **I oz. vodka**
- **juice of ½ lime**
- **I oz. cranberry juice**

Pour all of the ingredients in a cocktail shaker half-filled with ice. Cover, shake, and strain into a chilled martini glass.

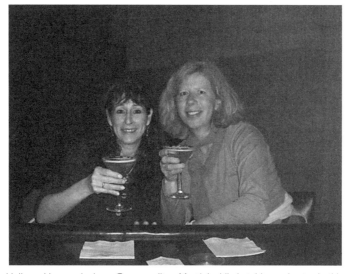

My friend Julia and I are enjoying a Cosmopolitan Martini while hatching a plan to do this regularly.

Martini Monday Strawberry Lemonade

My friend Sue made this for us one very hot and humid August day. It certainly hit the spot.

- **juice of 1 lemon**
- **1 tbsp. sugar**
- **8 to 10 ripe strawberries**
- **¾ cup water**
- **1½ oz. vodka**

Place all of the ingredients in a blender and blend until fairly smooth. Serve over ice.

Try the Chai

This martini is a bit different, but very tasty—so tasty that you may want to make a pitcher full!

- **2 oz. vodka**
- **2 oz. cold chai tea**
- **1 tsp. simple syrup**
- **2 tbsp. almond milk***
- **ground cinnamon for garnish**

Place the vodka, chai tea, simple syrup, and almond milk in a cocktail shaker over ice. Cover and shake until the outside of the shaker has frosted. Strain into a chilled martini glass and sprinkle with some ground cinnamon.

*Optional

Autumn Bliss

Here is a drink that really tastes like autumn. Garnish it with a cinnamon stick or some cinnamon heart candies.

- 1 oz. regular vodka or apple vodka
- 1 oz. cinnamon liqueur
- 2 oz. apple cider
- cinnamon stick or cinnamon heart candies for garnish

Fill a cocktail shaker with ice. Add the vodka, cinnamon liqueur, and cider. Shake vigorously to blend and chill. Strain into a martini glass. Allow the drink to clear before garnishing with the cinnamon stick or cinnamon heart candies and serving.

Sparkling Dream

If you are looking for a drink that is refreshing and has some fizz to it, try one (or two!) of these.

- 1 oz. pomegranate liqueur
- 1 oz. Cointreau
- 1 oz. fresh orange juice
- 3 oz. champagne or sparkling wine
- orange zest for garnish

Pour the pomegranate liqueur, Cointreau, and orange juice in a cocktail shaker over ice. Cover and shake to chill. Remove the lid and gently stir in the champagne. Pour into a martini glass and garnish with the orange zest.

The Christmas Grand-Cran

This beautiful crimson cocktail not only brings out the colour of the season, but a few of the favourite flavours. It is a delectable mix of Grand Marnier orange liqueur, cranberry, and rosemary and makes a stunning drink pairing for almost any holiday meal.

- 1 tsp. sugar
- 10 to 12 fresh rosemary needles
- 1 ½ oz. Grand Marnier
- 1 ½ oz. cranberry juice
- ½ oz. fresh lemon juice
- rosemary sprig for garnish

In a tall mixing glass, muddle the rosemary needles lightly with the sugar. Add the Grand Marnier, cranberry juice, lemon juice, and some ice cubes. Cover with the top of a cocktail shaker and shake vigorously. Strain over fresh ice into a rocks glass with ice. Garnish with a rosemary sprig.

Dirty Martini

I felt that it was necessary to include a recipe for a genuine martini. This one is very good. The olive juice tames down the gin just a little bit.

- 2 oz. gin
- 1 tbsp. dry vermouth
- 2 tbsp. olive juice
- 2 olives

Place all of the ingredients in a cocktail shaker and fill with ice. Cover and shake hard 3 to 4 times. Strain into a martini glass and add the olives.

THANK YOU!

Thank you to Mike Antolick for being the most patient husband ever.
Your wisdom and opinion are much appreciated and I think you are
the smartest and wisest man on earth.

Many thanks to Susan Williams who came up with the whole "Eat Well" idea.
I appreciate your faith in me and how you supported me, the business,
and then the cookbook. You are a good friend!

To Janice Harper for coming up with the great cookbook idea
and then supporting me continually.

I still have to pinch myself to believe that Terilee Bulger,
publisher of Acorn Press, was interested in publishing my cookbook.
What an honour! Thank you, Terrilee!

I'm a huge fan of very talented John Sylvester, so you can
imagine my excitement when he agreed to do the photo shoot.
He is as nice as he is talented. Thank you, John!

Thank you to Caitlin Drake who copy-edited the cookbook.
She has a good eye and lots of patience.

Many thanks to designer Matt Reid, who did fine work
on the design of the book and allowed me to use my vision.

Special thanks to my dad Con Zaat, for taking, keeping & gathering pictures.

Thank you to Perry Williams for coming to my rescue many times.

Thank you, Theresa…you are the wind beneath my wings!

To Elliot LaRonde and Yanet Roncal for testing,
tasting, and technical expertise. You two rock!

Special thanks to Gale Morgan who is always there for me.
Your friendship is most precious!

Thank you Sylvie Arsenault for the love and time you gave to this project.

To Margaret Flood for the amazing support, advice, and proofreading.
I'm so grateful!

Thank you Ellie Reddin for proof-reading, testing, and encouragement.

Many thanks to Nora Wotton for being such a great sport and coming
over at 5:30 in the morning and assisting the photographer.

I'm forever grateful to Rosemary Henderson for
so much more than I could possibly express.

Thank you to Charlie the Bookman for the tons of advice.

Thank you to Craig Mackie for your time and patience.

To Hans Anderegg, who is my culinary inspiration.
Thanks for showing me the way.

Many thanks to Georgia MacKenzie, Lorenda Maaskant,
and Liz Vaine for your guidance and recipes.

Special thanks to the Martini Monday Ladies for
everything you have done and continue to do.

Thank you to the Charlottetown Farmers' Market for getting me going.

And finally I want to express my sincere gratitude to all the wonderful
customers who supported me while I was getting started and over the
years, and to the many who became friends and shared their lives with me.
It is you who helped me keep a roof over my head. I feel so blessed to
have had those years to develop these relationships. I know I'm in
your thoughts and prayers as you are in mine.

INDEX